The Challenge of Person-Centred Care

An Interprofessional Perspective

Edited by

*Georgina Koubel, Department of Social Work,
Community and Mental Health, Canterbury Christ
Church University, UK
Hilary Bungay, Department of Allied Health,
Canterbury Christ Church University, UK*

palgrave
macmillan

First published 2009 by
PALGRAVE MACMILLAN

Palgrave Macmillan in the UK is an imprint of Macmillan Publishers Limited, registered in England, company number 785998, of Houndmills, Basingstoke, Hampshire RG21 6XS.

Palgrave Macmillan in the US is a division of St Martin's Press LLC, 175 Fifth Avenue, New York, NY 10010.

Palgrave Macmillan is the global academic imprint of the above companies and has companies and representatives throughout the world.

Palgrave® and Macmillan® are registered trademarks in the United States, the United Kingdom, Europe and other countries.

ISBN-13: 978–0–230–55077–3
ISBN-10: 0–230–550770

This book is printed on paper suitable for recycling and made from fully managed and sustained forest sources. Logging, pulping and manufacturing processes are expected to conform to the environmental regulations of the country of origin.

A catalogue record for this book is available from the British Library.

10 9 8 7 6 5 4 3 2 1
18 17 16 15 14 13 12 11 10 09

Printed and bound in China

Contents

Notes on Contributors

Jane Arnott is Senior Lecturer in Community Nursing in the Department of Social Work, Community and Mental Health at Canterbury Christ Church University. Jane has particular interests in developmental psychology and public health.

Claire Barber is Senior Lecturer in Mental Health in the Department of Social Work, Community and Mental Health at Canterbury Christ Church University. Her special interest is child and adolescent mental health.

Hilary Bungay is Senior Lecturer in Radiography in the Department of Allied Health at Canterbury Christ Church University, and has a part-time secondment as Senior Research Fellow in the Sidney de Haan Research Centre for Arts and Health. Her current research interests include the impact of music on health, older people and cancer services.

Tim Dunn is Senior Lecturer in Occupational Therapy in the Department of Allied Health at Canterbury Christ Church University. His special interests include areas of industrial wellness and health promotion through occupation.

Paul Elliott is Senior Lecturer in Nursing and Infection Control in the Department of Nursing and Applied Clinical Studies at Canterbury Christ Church University. He has primary research interests in psychosocial aspects of infection control, health psychology and person-centred development.

Laura Gilbert is Senior Lecturer in Child Nursing in the Department of Health, Well-Being and the Family at Canterbury Christ Church University.

Georgina Koubel is Senior Lecturer in Social Work in the Department of Social Work, Community and Mental Health at Canterbury Christ Church University. After working as a generic social worker in London for many years, Georgina moved to Kent Social Services where she worked in Adult Services while completing her MSc in Health and Community Studies. She has developed her work with older adults and adults with disabilities and takes a particular interest in the area of safeguarding vulnerable adults. She has also developed particular interests in interprofessional education, and collaborative and reflective practice.

Niall McLaughlin is Senior Lecturer in Mental Health in the Department of Social Work, Community and Mental Health at Canterbury Christ Church University. His special interest is in recovery in mental health and professional standards in mental health nursing.

Peter Milburn is Principal Lecturer in Radiography, and Campus Director of one of Canterbury Christ Church University's four campuses. His research interests include practitioner role development and the impact of interprofessional education on role redefinition and evolution within health and social care.

Rebecca Sandys is Senior Lecturer in Radiography at Canterbury Christ Church University. Her areas of interest include computerised tomography, forensic radiography and interprofessional working.

Patricia Walker is Senior Lecturer in Midwifery in the Department of Health, Well-Being and the Family at Canterbury Christ Church University.

Janet Wood is Senior Lecturer in Mental Health in the Department of Social Work, Community and Mental Health at Canterbury Christ Church University. Her special interests are in areas including partnership working, person-centred care practice, psychosocial interventions for psychosis and mental health nursing practice.

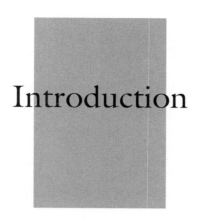

Introduction

Georgina Koubel and Hilary Bungay

If it is possible to identify one of the most significant developments in the health and social care environment in the past 20 years, it must be the move away from the 'professional agenda', which places the practitioner at the top of the apex of a triangle, where it is assumed that the doctor, nurse or social worker is the expert with all the power and knowledge, and the patient/client/service user along the base, as a passive recipient of professional wisdom. The crucial difference in the concept of person-centred care is that it requires practitioners to base their thinking and practice on the needs, wishes and rights of the person who is using health and social care services. This may be the way in which practitioners say they want to work or it may be quite a challenge for them, but it is not a matter of choice, as service users are now expected to be involved in the planning and prioritizing of service delivery and, according to Barrett *et al.* (2005: 15), 'The Government rhetoric promotes the principles of choice and control for service users within a seamless service'.

This reference to a 'seamless service' highlights the requirement for practitioners to move towards more collaboration and better communication between professionals. In response to this challenge some universities are offering professional training and education to health and social care practitioners in a setting that promotes learning and understanding in interprofessional groups.

This book emerged from discussions among a group of academics from a range of different professional backgrounds who were working together on one module on the Interprofessional Learning degree at Canterbury Christ Church University. The module was entitled Person-Centred Care and Interprofessional Collaboration and was offered to first-year students from eight pathways that made up the programme. These were students studying to become adult and child nurses, mental health nurses, midwives, social workers, occupational therapists, radiographers and operating department practitioners.

Although all of the staff members involved in developing and delivering the module were committed to the broad concept of interprofessional learning and the promotion of person-centred care, it soon became apparent when the team met that our understanding and interpretation of the issues were affected by the particular discipline from which each of us had come. In particular, the different perspectives of the nurses and the other groups made for some lively debates.

Issues of jargon and terminology were particularly difficult to disentangle. Even what we actually called the person or people on the receiving end of our services indicated a level of difference in the way we constructed our roles and understood our relationships. The medical practitioners spoke of 'patients' as if this were a generic term, but this did not fit with midwives highlighting 'women-centred care' or child nurses who saw their focus as the child and their family. Social workers talked of 'service users' and 'carers', while occupational therapists related to their 'clients'.

Trying to find a term that would please everyone became quite a challenge and in the end it was agreed that the only possible term we could all use was 'person'. Although this left room for ambiguity, it was felt that it avoided the profession-specific jargon that any of the other terms could imply. In this book, which has chapters written by a range of professionals, each writer has tried to use language that feels appropriate to him or her. However, throughout the book you will find that writers return to the question of language and how its use constructs the relationship between professional groups as well as with people who use services. A further aspect of the debate is whether we should call ourselves professionals or practitioners; neither of these concepts is uncontested and the only certainty is that no language can be completely value free. This is a continuing debate and one that informs our understanding of interprofessional working as well as the role and construction of those who deliver care and those in receipt of services. The ways in which we address these issues are fundamental to the discussions around how we work together.

> If one of the purposes of interprofessional working is the combining of different perspectives then the patients or service users are interprofessional workers par excellence as in the vast majority of cases it is they… who unify and combine the different advice and perspectives integrating them into daily living and making health choices as they do so.
>
> (Ovretveit *et al.* 1997: 117)

In order to gain a better understanding of each other's perspectives, it was important that we were able to factor in discussions about the commonalities and differences between our views around our relationships with people who received services and with each other. This involved discussion of the values and attitudes that we had developed as professionals from different disciplines. One of the key factors that drew us together was a common concern for individuals and a commitment to the notion of ensuring that people were treated with dignity and respect. In this sense our values were largely consistent, and focus on our understanding of the rights and autonomy of individuals who access health and social care. However, in terms of constructing our *relationships* with people who used services there were a range of views, from the 'medical expert' model that says that the professional knows what is best for their patients to a 'social model' that constructs the barriers to achievement for individuals in the social realm rather than according to the impairment of the individual.

> The different philosophies of care underpinning these two orientations – the medical and social models – have consistently posed dilemmas in our understanding and differentiation of care. The dominance in the medical profession in the arena of care has led to inappropriate medicalization of social problems tying people into a dependency relationship.
>
> (Philips 2007: 128)

Human rights, ethical frameworks and the values that inform professional practice and the ways in which they are applied can make a great deal of difference to the experience of someone who is in need of services. The social model of care identifies issues of power in the professional role (Thompson 2007) and looks at how the 'helping' relationship can also prove to be disempowering and produce a level of dependency on the professional (Shakespeare 2000). Person-centred care encompasses this model, therefore the issue of power and its impact on interprofessional working is another theme that is revisited in a number of the chapters.

This book is committed to helping readers explore the dilemmas and navigate the maze of interprofessional person-centred care. The exercises will help you in finding routes that can encompass diverse views and address the range of perspectives, while also keeping the person at the centre of our considerations. In order to question practices and procedures that may be taken for granted if they do not genuinely include the rights and needs of people in health and social care, we have to be able to reflect, question and try to understand ourselves (Jasper 2006) as people and practitioners, as well as gaining a working knowledge of the complex climate that operates in contemporary health and social care.

Although interprofessional working is not a new concept, it does seem to be an idea whose time has come. Collaborative working has many supporters and anyone who has worked with colleagues from diverse disciplines will know what can be achieved when a vision of person-centred care informs the aims and goals of all the practitioners involved (Braye & Preston-Shoot 1995). Nevertheless, respecting and valuing the views and expertise of others, including that of the service user, rather than promoting the superiority of one's own profession still presents organisational and interpersonal challenges. The requirement for practitioners from health and social care to understand and interprofessional working and person-centred care entails engagement with different ways of working and involves seeing the world from a range of perspectives rather than maintaining the comfort of a familiar, profession-specific spotlight on the world. However, this emphasis on interprofessional working also requires a significant reorientation of professional working practices (Barrett *et al.* 2005).

Awareness of the psychological factors at work in both organisational and interpersonal relationships can help to conceptualise the benefits of and, importantly, some of the barriers to effective person-centred care or interprofessional collaboration. Obholzer and Roberts (1994) highlight from a psychodynamic perspective the challenges that arise for practitioners who are working with issues that are highly emotionally charged, and the sometimes destructive strategies that teams can put in place to cope with the feelings and personal pressures that can arise from care work.

While there is a risk that academic psychology can provide too deterministic an approach to sit comfortably with the craft of recognising the individual worth of each person and engaging with them on that basis, the application of some models such as the phenomenological or humanist approach developed by Carl Rogers (cited in Nicolson *et al.* 2006) does address many of the principles and values that underlie person-centred care. Throughout the chapters the authors in this book return regularly to the values and attitudes that are so important if person-centred care is to achieve the transition from government rhetoric to the reality of experience for those who use health and social care services.

Equally, person-centred care cannot operate in a context that does not take into account the social structures and interpersonal elements that affect the lives of service users, carers and practitioners. In order to promote the individual rights and needs of service users, practitioners also have to understand how person-centred practice takes into account elements such as class, culture, ethnicity, age, gender and sexuality. Anti-discriminatory practice is therefore crucial in providing a context that underpins a number of the challenges for practitioners who are trying to promote empowering practice (Thompson 2007). Person-centred care and interprofessional practice both need to factor in issues such as racism, sexism and ageism so that practitioners have the sensitivity and understanding to ensure that individuals who access health and social care services stay at the heart of relationships with service users and colleagues.

Practitioners working in health and social care are more than aware of the challenges that the government's agenda holds for them, where change seems to be the only constant. However, respect for those who use services and promoting their ability to have an impact on how those services are delivered will enhance the work of practitioners and benefit both in the long run. While more equal relationships among practitioners from diverse disciplines and between practitioners and service users can provide a better environment for practice, collaborative, person-centred practice will not develop by itself. This book therefore looks at a range of perspectives that inform areas of special interest in health and social work and uses these to develop a conceptual framework for practitioners and students who are trying to engage with the benefits and challenges of person-centred, interprofessional care.

People enter employment in the health and social care services for a variety of reasons and motivations, and these, in conjunction with their own personal circumstances, will influence how they practise and collaborate with colleagues from other disciplines. Similarly, the personal circumstances and previous experiences of those accessing services will affect how they perceive and respond to practitioners. Despite recent scandals such as GP Harold Shipman's conviction as a serial murderer and the Bristol Royal Infirmary Inquiry into death rates in paediatric cardiac surgery, there is evidence that trust in medical and health care practitioners remains high. Calnan and Sandford (2004) found that people's trust in services is influenced by the extent to which the doctor appears patient centred and the perceived level of professional expertise. Whether care is described as patient centred or person centred, the most important issue is trust, because for people to engage with treatment or interventions they need to have trust in the practitioner providing the service.

In order to help readers to understand and reflect on the issues that inform person-centred care and interprofessional working, the book contains a series of case studies and reflective exercises that we have called *challenges*. Whether you are a first-year student who is looking at some of these issues for the first time or a practitioner revisiting some of the concepts in the book and reviewing your own attitudes and experiences, you will benefit from time spent thinking about the questions that are asked and developing your understanding of the value and application of the concepts.

Plan of the book

This book is organised into eight chapters and arranged in three parts. Part I (Chapters 1 and 2) provides an introduction to person-centred care and interprofessional working in the context of health and social care. Part II (Chapters 3, 4 and 5) looks at the theory and ethics of person-centred care and interprofessional working, and Part III (Chapters 6, 7 and 8) applies the theory to areas of practice; health promotion, adult protection and carers. However, it is clearly recognised that it is the *integration* of theoretical frameworks into practice that will enhance person-centred interprofessional care, and the chapters contain a number of examples that can be used to help you to think about how the more abstract ideas can inform your thinking, planning and the process of practice.

In Chapter 1, Milburn and Walker examine the shift from patient- to person-centred care in the context of the evolution of the health and social care services. A definition of interprofessional working is provided, which clarifies the potential confusion that has arisen due to changes of terminology from 'multi' to 'inter' over recent years. There then follows a critical debate covering the development of interprofessional education and collaborative practice and deliberating on how interprofessional practice can support person-centred care in the care setting. By the end of the chapter it is hoped that the reader has a clear understanding of how person-centred care and interprofessional working are intrinsically linked.

Elliott and Koubel in Chapter 2 consider the meaning of the concept of person-centred care, and explore its origins in relation to interprofessional working and good practice in the current climate of health and social care. There is consideration of theoretical and value frameworks that inform person-centred care and a series of challenges aiming to develop your ability to reflect on the concept of person-centred care and the importance of adopting a holistic, anti-discriminatory perspective when working with people.

In Chapter 3, Bungay and Sandys, explore the notion of 'What is a person?' in the belief that we cannot practise person-centred care without some common understanding of personhood. Similarly, although much of recent government policy refers to person-centred care and the need to treat people with dignity and respect, these too are abstract terms. Do we really know what dignity means and does it mean the same to all people? Throughout this chapter there are a number of case studies designed to assist you in drawing your own conclusions and definitions on what a person is. When does someone become a person or stop being a person? What does it mean to treat someone with dignity and respect?

In Chapter 4, Barber, McLaughlin and Wood introduce the idea that it is crucial for practitioners to have self-awareness to be able to practise in a person-centred manner. They suggest that our verbal and non-verbal communication skills are influenced by both culturally entrenched professional 'norms' and our own values, which consciously and unconsciously affect our perceptions of others. To help increase self-awareness the authors offer the Johari window as a model to enable readers to question their beliefs and perceptions of others and how these affect care delivery.

In Chapter 5, Arnott presents the argument that an individual's 'moral intuition' is not sufficient to meet the challenges of day-to-day health and social care, and that practitioners need to have some knowledge of an ethical framework to underpin their practice. She uses ethical theories that have informed health and social care practice, such as consequentialism, deotonology and virtue ethics. Exploring the development of human rights, she reflects on the relationship between the roles and responsibilities of care professionals and the rights of the patient or client.

Gilbert and Dunn in Chapter 6 look at what health promotion means for health and social care practice and discuss the different strategies that can be used for the person-centred delivery of health promotion. A narrative approach facilitates the understanding of the roles of different professionals in empowering individuals and communities to improve their health. The authors also question some of the possible variables influencing how individuals or communities may or may not be able to, or may choose not to, prioritise a particular health issue as a key concern to address, and identify the factors that help or hinder the delivery of person-centred health promotion.

In Chapter 7, Koubel weighs up the attitudes and values found in adult protection, and explores the perception of who is a vulnerable adult and what makes people vulnerable. She identifies what abuse is and how signs and symptoms can be recognised, using case studies to help the reader consider the legal and ethical issues arising in response to safeguarding adults. Koubel challenges us as to how we can maintain an empowering, person-centred perspective while promoting appropriate interprofessional working in relation to developing effective practice in safeguarding vulnerable adults. She further asks us to reflect on the differences and similarities between child and adult protection and the lessons we can learn from child protection.

In Chapter 8, Bungay and Walker consider the distinct input made by carers and practitioners to care, and review the support mechanisms in place for carers and practitioners in the context of institutional and community provision. Potential conflicts exist between the care recipient, the carer and practitioners because of the nature of the caring relationship. The authors reflect on the possible causes of these conflicts and the importance of collaboration between all those concerned.

Each chapter can be read as a stand-alone piece of work, however throughout the book common themes emerge, for example the issues of human rights, communication, empowerment, dignity and respect. These are all central to person-centred care and effective interprofessional working.

References

Barrett, G., Selman, D. & Thomas, G. (2005) *Interprofessional Working in Health and Social Care: Professional Perspectives.* Basingstoke: Palgrave Macmillan.

Braye, S. & Preston-Shoot, M. (1995) *Empowering Practice in Social Care.* Buckingham: Open University Press.

Calnan, M. & Sandford, E. (2004) Public trust in health care: The system or the doctor? *Quality and Safety in Health Care,* 13: 92–7.

Jasper, M. (2006) *Professional Development, Reflection and Decision Making.* Oxford: Blackwell.

Nicolson, P., Bayne, R. & Owen, J. (2006) *Applied Psychology for Social Workers,* 3rd edn. Basingstoke: Palgrave Macmillan.

Obholzer, A. & Roberts, V. Z. (1994) *The Unconscious at Work: Stress in the Human Services.* London: Routledge.

Ovretveit, J., Mathias, P. & Thompson, T. (1997) *Interprofessional Working for Health and Social Care.* Basingstoke: Macmillan.

Philips, J. (2007) *Care.* Cambridge: Polity Press.

Shakespeare, T. (2000) *Help.* Birmingham: Venture Press.

Thompson, N. (2007) *Power and Empowerment.* Lyme Regis: Random House.

An Introduction to Person-Centred Care and Interprofessional Working

Beyond Interprofessional Education and towards Collaborative Person-Centred Practice

Peter Milburn and Pat Walker

This book seeks to investigate the concept of person-centred care within the context of interprofesssional care delivery. We start by considering the evolution of person-centred care in health and social care, and explores the development of interprofessional education and its contribution to collaborative person-centred care.

This chapter challenges you to:

- Consider how the concept of person-centred care emerged.

- Explore the meanings of interprofessional working.

- Critically evaluate the impact of interprofessional education on health and social care practice.

- Consider 'life after interprofessional education' – could this be collaborative person-centred care?

- Consider how collaborative person-centred care can be achieved.

Evolution of person-centred care in the context of health and social care

During the nineteenth century there was little that the medical profession or the limited available health care provision could do in terms of curing disease and the causes of ill health, and the most effective interventions for the health of the nation were public health measures that improved sanitation and urban living conditions. Concern about questions of social welfare and policy grew throughout the nineteenth century, as the Industrial Revolution saw the movement of people away from traditional rural economies to more prosperous cities. Issues of child labour, extreme poverty, crime and squalor were reflected in the works of novelists such as Charles Dickens and research undertaken by philanthropists such as Lord Shaftesbury and Seebohm Rowntree (Blakemore 2003). One of the major players in the promotion of modern social care and social work was Octavia Hill, who set up an organisation to manage rented properties allocated to 'deserving' families. Middle-class volunteers (usually women who traditionally did not go into paid employment) would collect the rents, and provide advice and 'casework' to the poor families who benefited from the scheme. Hill then became a key founder of the Charity Organisation Society, which provided an early organisational base for social work.

Towards the end of the nineteenth century the state became more involved in the provision of health and welfare, and medicine advanced as a science. As this happened the medical model of health became prominent, focusing on the individual cause of illness and the search for specific individual cures (Ham 1992). As a result, the individualistic concept of health became dominant, and economic and social causes of ill health were overshadowed.

However the late nineteenth and early twentieth centuries also saw the emergence of a political group who were committed to notions of citizenship and equality, and whose analysis of society was that the problems encountered by the working classes were not because of their inherent character flaws, which could only be addressed through casework and moral guidance, but were the result of structural inequalities that could be ameliorated by changing society and providing equal opportunities for everyone.'

The ideas of the Labour Party informed much of the legislation that sought to provide for a more equal society, particularly after the Second World War when the Party was voted into power with a large majority and, based on the principles outlined in the Beveridge Report (1942), set about establishing a welfare state that gave people rights to services such as medical care, housing, education, employment and personal social services. One of Labour's major initiatives was the National Health Service (NHS), which came into being in 1948 on the founding principles of collectivism, comprehensiveness, equality and universality (Allsop 1995). However, the emphasis was on the provision of personal medical services, and doctors had a decisive role in determining the nature of services. Allsop (*ibid.*) believes that the organisation of services was strongly influenced by the division of labour in health services at the time, as well as by the history of state intervention during the nineteenth and twentieth centuries.

The power and status that the medical profession gained during the twentieth century meant that doctors were held in high esteem. When someone attended an appointment with a medical practitioner the consultation was 'doctor centred'; that is, the doctor led the encounter using direct and closed questioning and giving the patient instructions and directions (Byrne & Long 1976 in Mead & Bower 2000). The problem is that even in acute hospital settings, people attending appointments may have chronic conditions or disabilities but would describe themselves as healthy and not consider themselves to be ill or a 'patient', yet they are labelled as such by the system. Some terms are so embedded in our professional language that we fail even to think about how their meaning could reduce the individuality of the person concerned. In medical settings, the person who needs services is habitually referred to as a patient without any real consideration of the meaning of the term. Yet in ancient Latin the word from which patient derives, *patior*, means to suffer (Neuberger & Tallis 1999), and one of the definitions of patient in the *Oxford English Dictionary* is 'able to wait without becoming annoyed or anxious'.

The term 'patient' is generally taken to imply illness, infirmity, incapacity or incapability. Therefore use of the word may be perceived as presenting a negative stereotype that is not consistent with the concept of person-centred care as set out by Price (2006), who defines it as a process of involvement, individuality and understanding. The model of person-centred care needs to encompass the idea of a person's strengths, choices and rights as well as their needs and vulnerabilities. However, the term patient fails to reflect any of this and its use is inconsistent with a person-centred perspective.

Within the context of social care, use of the term 'client' is also a stereotype that, like patient, may have negative connotations. Client comes from the Latin *cliens*, a variant of *cluens* meaning 'heeding', and originally denoted a person under the protection or patronage of another. Thus, like the term patient in relation to the health professional (that is, a passive recipient of professional expertise), the idea of clienthood in relation to social work is a concept constructed to represent a certain kind of relationship, which can usually be categorised in terms of the unequal power relationship between the role of client and that of worker (Payne 1997). Equally, the term 'user', which appears in more common parlance today, may be commonly associated with the concept of people who abuse drugs or a person who manipulates others for their own gain. Despite this, 'service user' has been identified as the least discriminatory term available and is currently used extensively. But none of these terms is truly consistent with the concept of person-centred care, as each has a measure of dependency or need associated with it and could be construed negatively if the literal definitions are accepted. On the other hand, using 'person' is appropriate as it is a neutral term in the sense that it can be applied to people who are accessing both health and social services, has no negative associations and is non-judgemental.

Person-centred care was introduced as a concept in psychotherapy and counselling by Carl Rogers in 1961. However, at this time in the health literature the phrase 'patient-centred care' was starting to appear and since the late 1960s there has been an extensive body of literature advocating the patient-centred approach to medical care. For example, Balint (1969) described patient-centred medicine as understanding the patient as a unique human being, and McWhinney (1989) suggested that the physician should try to enter the patient's world to see the illness through the patient's eyes. In 2002, Coulter described the essence of patient-centred care as involving and informing patients; responding quickly and effectively to patient needs and wishes;

and ensuring patients are treated in a dignified and supportive manner. She suggests that only patients know about their experience of illness, their social circumstances, their preferences and their attitudes to risk, and in doing so supports the position of the Bristol Inquiry (Kennedy 2001) that patients should be treated as equals with different levels of expertise.

A number of ongoing government initiatives have been launched since the 1990s aiming to place patients at centre stage. The Patient's Charter (Department of Health 1991), for instance, attempted to pursue a more consumer-led approach to health care and introduced certain measures such as reducing waiting times in outpatient clinics in a move towards a more patient-oriented NHS (Bury 1997). Thus we can see that there has been a gradual paradigm shift from doctor-centred to patient-centred care, with political moves to make the service more patient oriented. A further shift took place in 2000, when the phrase 'person-centred care' started appearing in policy documents; see for example *The NHS Plan* (Department of Health 2000), *National Service Framework for Older People* (Department of Health 2001a) or *Valuing People* (Department of Health 2001b). Person-centred care has been defined as enabling independence, choice, inclusion, equality or empowerment (Dowling *et al.* 2006). It is worth taking a moment to consider the similarities and differences between this and Coulter's perspective on patient-centred care.

CHALLENGE

■ What do you think the differences are between patient-centred care and person-centred care?

■ Why do you think there is a difference?

■ Would you prefer to be treated in a patient-centred or a person-centred manner?

The NHS Plan (DH 2000) agenda was intended to bring a fundamental change in health and social care delivery. This involved a cultural shift to design and deliver services around the person and their needs, not the needs of the organisation. There was a shift in the balance of power from professional to patient (DH 2001c), which recognised patients as experts in their own right in their knowledge and understanding, especially if they had a chronic health problem (DH 2001d). Another direction involved the person's responsibility for their own health through the adoption of a healthy lifestyle and responsible use of available services. Over the following years new service commitments within the NHS Plan were introduced to enhance flexible and efficient service access via NHS Direct and walk-in centres.

This consumer approach to health care means in theory that patients are no longer seen as passive recipients of care, but as being empowered. User involvement is encouraged, as is the notion of the 'expert patient'. Patients are seen as 'active consumers' with rights to certain standards of treatment, to full information, and to be treated with respect and actively involved in decision making about their care. Some authors argue that the government has a limited understanding of the intricacy of person-centredness for staff involved in care (Dewing 2004). However, irrespective of whether person-centred care is viewed as idealistic, practitioners are required to translate the concept into practice and evaluate its delivery.

The philosophy of patient and professional involvement in care decisions and provision has grown over recent years, with a strengthening desire to build trust between service users and providers, improve standards of care and shift the balance of power. Such values exist not only at operational levels but also at intermediate and strategic levels of health care provision. Government policy places a greater emphasis on personal patient circumstances, patient diversity and care tailored to individual needs and wants in a more personalised, integrated process of care provision. 'Integrating care is a key driver of personalisation' (DH 2007a: 32).

In *Our NHS, Our Future: NHS Next Stage Review* there was great emphasis on the centrality of person-centred care that is organised and systematic, with the traditional boundaries of primary and secondary care provision becoming redundant through improved integrated service provision (DH 2007a). To date, interprofessional education to support integrated care and greater interprofessional awareness has had a mixed reception. Some have identified resistance to interprofessional working (Dalton *et al.* 2003; Reeves 2000, 2001); conversely, staff surveys suggest a willingness and preference for collaborative input in care provision (DH 2007b). Existing governmental support for integrated care requires educational services to develop interprofessional education even further, with improved implementation to build integrity in the theory and practice areas of course provision at undergraduate and continuing professional education levels.

Person-centred care and interprofessional working

The development of health and social care services is significant in relation to person-centred care and indeed interprofessional working. The early emphasis on curative medicine and acute services placed the individual patient at the centre in the care of a doctor. In terms of professionals working together in the NHS, doctors were (and some would say still are) the most dominant and powerful group and other disciplines, for example nurses, radiographers and therapists, were always in subservient roles (see Witz 1992 for a comprehensive analysis of power in the health care professions). Such a relationship does not foster the concept of interprofessional working. Similarly, when we look at how the funding from central government has been allocated between health and social services, and indeed between different elements of each service, they have had to compete for limited resources. Today's health and social care workforce work together in ways that would never have been anticipated in the past, with different groups extending and expanding their roles. Some disciplines in the NHS and social services are now regularly meeting, and collaborating, with people from disciplines that they never would have had contact with in the past. This brings new challenges to individuals and their professional bodies and their educators to ensure effective working.

Consider the challenges of interprofessional working for:

■ Individual practitioners.

■ Professional bodies or trade unions.

■ Education.

Person-centred care as a concept and basis for care provision is dependent on interpretation at operational level in institutional and community care settings. However, significant intermediate managerial and strategic issues do arise, with the involvement of various stakeholders, including educational providers. According to the Royal College of Nursing (2004), implementation of person-centred care will require two fundamental changes in health care delivery: a different style of interaction and alternative ways of organising health care delivery and systems. Extensive educational development at undergraduate and postgraduate level will be needed to achieve collaborative person-centred care

The issue of terminology has for many years proved a problematic area for the 'interprofessional' movement; and so a brief consideration of the different terms follows. Terms in current usage include multiprofessional, interprofessional, multidisciplinary, interdisciplinary, multi-agency and interagency.

'Multi' generally means the involvement of people from different professions, for example multidisciplinary teams (MDTs) are commonly found in cancer care. MDTs consist of all disciplines concerned in the diagnosis and treatment of a specific cancer type, for example recto-colon cancer or breast cancer. These teams usually meet on a weekly basis and are represented by a member of each discipline involved in the care pathway (including radiographer, radiologist, surgeon, oncologist, specialist nurse and histopathologist). Each case is discussed and each team member shares their expertise and knowledge. This includes the input of the specialist nurse, who may well have knowledge of the patient's social and psychological aspects. Together the team decides the best possible options that may be offered to the patient. The advantages of such a process are the correlation between clinical, imaging and cytological/histological findings during the discussion, that decisions can be discussed and questioned from a broad base of knowledge, and that the presence of all those involved in a person's diagnosis and treatment should ensure that the patient receives consistent information and coordinated treatment (Improving Outcomes in Breast Cancer 1996). This can be reassuring for patients when they know that a number of experts have considered the treatment options available to them. The staff involved in such a process also report a positive view, as some feel that it raises intellectual standards and that working with other experts makes it enjoyable. They also feel supported in agreeing treatment with others (Bungay 2001).

'Inter', on the other hand, suggests collaboration, particularly in areas of decision making (Pollard *et al.* 2005). It can therefore be tricky to distinguish between the two terms, because it appears it would be difficult for multiprofessionals or multidisciplinary teams to work together without interacting or collaborating. However, a person may have a number of different agencies involved in their care and so be receiving multi-agency and multiprofessional care without the different agencies communicating directly. Although this seems confusing, looking at Leathard's (1994) work can help to clarify the terminology. She suggests that these terms in common use have clear distinctions, and if such distinctions are recognised and understood our awareness of the processes at work will be clearer too. For Leathard, terms such as 'interprofessional', 'multiprofessional', 'interdisciplinary', 'multidisciplinary', 'transprofessional', 'transdisciplinary', 'holistic' and 'generic' are concept-based terms – that is, terms that have as their underlying structure a concept or ideology – whereas terms such as 'shared learning', 'group work', 'cross-agency', 'intersectoral agency', 'joint working' and 'common core' are process-based terms – in other words, terms that seek to describe a process, event or action that is occurring.

For the purposes of this book the following definition will be adopted: Interprofessional working means collaborative practice, 'that is the process whereby members of different professions and/or agencies work together to provide integrated health and/or social care for the benefit of the service user' (Pollard *et al.* 2005: 10).

Although this may seem obvious and straightforward, in reality there are barriers to effective collaborative practice. Each professional group has evolved through history with its own knowledge base, values and attitudes, and professional culture. There also exists a professional hierarchy within the health and social care systems. For example, in the case of the MDTs described above, the leader of the teams is generally a surgeon or oncologist rather than a nurse specialist or radiographer. The traditional organisation of health and social care workers' education has produced individuals who are socialised into their own professional culture with its associated language, terminology and world view, who see their patients/clients/service users from a particular and limited perspective without considering the broader context of the person involved. To work in a person-centred manner, professionals need to work collaboratively. This means maintaining profession-specific roles but being able to work together as a team so that 'they identify and analyze problems, define goals and assume joint responsibility for actions and interventions' (Counsell *et al.* 1999 in Hall 2005: 192). However, in order to achieve this team members must have an understanding of others' capabilities and roles. One way for health and social care practitioners to develop the necessary collaborative skills is for them to be given the opportunity to learn together (Hall 2005). In recognition of this there has been a move towards interprofessional education programmes.

Interprofessional education and interprofessional working

In the following sections the historical context for the development of interprofessional education (IPE) is considered, raising questions and debate as to how and why the 'IPE movement' gathered pace during the late 1990s and for the first time had an impact on the design, delivery and organisation of undergraduate, pre-registration curricula. This and subsequent chapters will draw on the significant experience gained by staff at Canterbury Christ Church University through the development of a Master's framework in interprofessional education during the 1990s, and in the early years of the twenty-first century extending this expertise to major undergraduate provision. The collaborative initiative brought together for the first time students, practice staff, academic staff, professional bodies and the statutory and regulatory organisations across professional health and social care disciplines and supported the introduction of an interprofessional programme that involved all areas of the faculty of Health and Social Care.

Bringing together different professions to learn alongside and with one another is not a new idea, but despite the now considerable history of IPE, there remains debate around how to recognise its success or otherwise (Baldwin 1996; Barr 2000, 2002; Leathard 1994; Szasz 1969). It is argued that interprofessional education represents an educational model, a learning and teaching strategy that has as its goal bringing about effective interprofessional collaborative working; interprofessional education is a 'means to an end', not an end in itself. The debate must move on from 'deliverability' and the practicalities of timetabling and scheduling to a discussion focusing on interprofessional, person-centred collaborative practice and how the user will benefit from a service built and delivered by practitioners understanding and working interprofessionally. It is suggested that the beneficial impact of interprofessional education will be witnessed in practitioners delivering care that is wholly 'person centred' – care that achieves a balance of highly developed professional skill and expertise delivered within the a framework of individualised, person-centred need.

The World Health Organisation suggests that the terms 'interprofessional' and 'multiprofessional' are equivalent and interchangeable (WHO 1987) and defines multiprofessional as:

> the process by which a group of students (or workers) from the health related occupations with different educational backgrounds learn together during certain periods of their education, with interaction as an important goal, to collaborate in providing promotive, preventative, rehabilitative and other health related services.
>
> (WHO 1987: 6)

For others, interprofessional and multiprofessional represent clear distinctions in the *learning* models in place (O'Halloran *et al.* 2006). Barr (cited in *ibid.*), while accepting the WHO definition of multiprofessional, would call the activity interprofessional learning, seeing multiprofessional education as an all-encompassing term used to describe the 'ever-widening spread of learning opportunities which embrace more than one profession' (Barr 1994: 105). Interestingly however, while we accept that classification is an important part of any scientific endeavour, elaborating a typology consisting of lots of neatly labelled boxes will not necessarily tell us very much about interprofessionalism as a whole. The act of definition is not politically neutral, and excessively tight definitions can have serious consequences for collaborative practice (Trevillion & Bedford 2003). Too narrow definitions of interprofessionalism, which focus only on powerful professional interests and ignore service users, can 'become an additional barrier to user participation' (Biggs 1993: 156 cited in Trevillion & Bedford 2003). Trevillion and Bedford go on to suggest that fragmentation is not the only problem: conventional typologies tend to prioritise form and structure over content and process, running the risk of producing overly abstract descriptions that fail to capture the experience of interprofessionalism. The real debate perhaps needs to focus on what proactive, interactive learning needs to encourage; what will facilitate effective, collaborative service delivery in the practice setting; and what skills, knowledge and understanding practitioners require about their own and others' professional practice to deliver efficient, effective, person-centred care. Having gained this understanding, the next stage of identifying what, how and when such understanding and knowledge can best be gained will inform curriculum development around more precisely understood practice outcomes.

Humphris and Clark (2007: 59) present a useful curriculum model (Facilitated Collaborative Interprofessional Learning) that links three models of learning – guided discovery learning, collaborative learning and interprofessional learning – as a means to assist students in recognising their own and other professionals' contribution and role within a practice team. The model, rooted in experiential learning and delivered in both university and practice settings, seeks to identify collaborative skills that facilitate collaborative practice. Similarly, Colyer and Smith (2008) developed a work-based Collaborative Practice module that, through using action learning sets and an assessment strategy based on a patchwork text, aims to assist learners in identifying the collaborative learning skills essential for collaborative practice. As described by Colyer and Smith, action learning is a facilitated process of review and reflection that brings students together in small groups to undertake specific learning activities centred on the following themes: roles and boundaries; respect, trust and power; conflict and difference. The sets are facilitated by members of academic or clinical staff with the purpose of developing the students' understanding and knowledge around the selected themes. The chosen form of assessment, the 'patchwork text', is an integral part of the module (Crow *et al.* 2005). Students are asked to compose three short pieces of written work around each of the action learning set themes. These patches of text are used to simulate debate and discussion within the action learning sets and, together with a final patch of text, the collective 'stitch' together forms an individualised account of the student's experience of engagement with collaborative practice.

A changed way of thinking: collaborative person-centred care

The aim of a health and social care service is to develop and deliver structured support shaped around the needs of individual service users, their families and the community within which they live. Interprofessional education has been adopted (and interestingly interpreted very differently) by universities as the educational curriculum framework of choice to equip practitioners with the necessary professional and collaborative knowledge and skills to deliver the required service. As to whether the practice of bringing student groups together in whatever curriculum structure the university has chosen to validate (normally, however, under the banner of IPE) will achieve, or is achieving, the required goal will need to be measured against clearly defined practice outcomes: namely the ability of highly skilled practitioners to deliver a complex set of professional skills in close and meaningful collaboration with relevant colleagues and positioning the client at the centre of the service, thus achieving collaborative person-centred care.

What is collaborative person-centred practice?

Collaborative person-centred practice (CPCP), brought about through interprofessional education, involves the continuous interaction of two or more professions organised into common effort, to solve or explore common issues with the best possible participation of the patient (Curran 2004). Three components of effective collaborative person-centred care can be identified: continuous interaction, organised common effort and acceptance of the participation of the user:

- *Continuous interaction* is care organised in a way that provides continuity of care through collaborative interaction between the practitioners, the user and their family.

- *Organised common effort* is based on the premise and acceptance that no one profession can provide all the care needs for the user and that the organisational management of effort is critical in ensuring that the 'person' remains at the centre of activity.

- *Acceptance that the participation of the user* must be at the centre of care and an integral part of the decision-making process leads to the definition of a successful expected outcome.

Collaborative person-centred practice is designed to promote the active participation of each discipline in the delivery of care and, through such collaboration, to enhance patient- and family-centred goals and values. CPCP also provides mechanisms for continuous communication among care givers and in doing so optimises practitioner and client participation in clinical decision making within and across disciplines (Canadian Institute for Health Information 2003). Collaborative person-centred care is about developing a care system that maximises efficiency by recognising professional similarities and differences and promoting effective and efficient 'across boundaries' working, as opposed to pursuing a policy that seeks to 'blur professional boundaries'. This latter approach opportunistically extends the scope of professional practice and creates the potential risk of introducing 'system gaps' through which the more vulnerable people in our society may fall.

The effective delivery of collaborative person-centred practice requires confident, competent practitioners, highly skilled within their own area of professional practice, who possess a clear working knowledge, understand their own and others' practice boundaries and, above all, have sufficient knowledge to collaborate and communicate efficiently across boundaries to ensure that the 'system gaps' do not appear. The reward is a system of care that 'enhances patient – and family – centred goals and values, provides mechanisms for continues communication amongst caregivers, optimises staff participation in clinical decisions-making within and across disciplines, and fosters respect for the disciplinary contributions of all professionals' (Curran 2004).

Achieving collaborative person-centred care through interprofessional education

Programmes of interprofessional education in the UK, the US and Canada have evolved since the late 1990s (Cleghorn and Baker 2000; Gelmon *et al*. 2000). In the UK initiatives such as the Department of Health-funded New Generation Project provided an opportunity for pre-registration students to learn and work alongside one another, with the aim of enhancing professional collaboration and teamwork skills and thus realising an improved quality of care (O'Halloran *et al*. 2006).

This section examines the evidence suggesting that collaborative person-centred care can be achieved more effectively through interprofessional programmes by considering factors driving the need for a 'new generation' of health and social care practitioners. Is there a common philosophical value base that underpins IPE? What, if any, are the agreed core requirements for interprofessional programmes? What of the evidence base that supports the supposition that interprofessional education enhances interprofessional working? Are we witnessing a fundamental change in the culture of both the practice and preparation for practice of the health and social care professions?

The precise moment at which new initiatives commence is often difficult to identify, and this is no less the case for IPE. Research in the US suggests that interest in interprofessional education can be traced back to the late 1960s (Szasz, 1969). The first coordinated federal initiative was started in 1994 by the Institute for Health Improvement, supported by the Pew Health Professions Commission and the Bureau of Health Professions (see Cleghorn and Baker 2000; Gelmon *et al*. 2000 in Wilcock and Headrick 2000; Knapp *et al*. 2000). In the UK, the first evidence of coordinated interest in IPE can be identified by the formation of the Centre for the Advancement of Interprofessional Education in 1987, an organisation acting as a focus for research relating to IPE for the UK statutory, voluntary and independent sectors. The first major UK government initiative was the New Generation Project, recognised as a 'leading-edge site' to take forward common learning in 2002 (O'Halloran *et al*. 2006).

There is some consensus across the UK, US and Canada that IPE initiatives have common aims, aspirations and assumptions, namely:

- The promotion of interprofessional collaborative working among health and social care professionals.

- All aspects of curriculum design and delivery facilitate interactive learning between professional groups.

- The curriculum content is designed to enable students to develop the relevant knowledge and understanding of other professions that will facilitate effective interprofessional working and collaborative person-centred practice.

- The programme both encourages and provides progressive opportunities for professionals to learn with, from and about one another, to ensure respect for the integrity and contributions of others (adapted from Parsell and Bligh 1998).

As importantly, 'interdisciplinary education competencies' have been suggested for the domains of knowledge, skills and attitudes that could be used by practitioners to assess effective interprofessional working. Possible indicators of 'professional competence' for a practitioner working interprofessionally could be that such a practitioner would be able to:

- Describe their roles and responsibilities clearly to other professions.

- Recognise and observe the constraints of their role, responsibilities and competence, yet perceive the needs of patients/clients in a wider framework.

- Recognise and respect the role, responsibilities and competence of other professions in relation to their own role.

- Work with other professions to effect change and resolve conflict in the provision of care and treatment.

- Work with others to assess, plan, provide and review care for individual patients.

- Tolerate difference, misunderstanding and shortcomings in other professions.

- Facilitate interprofessional case conference and team meetings.

- Enter into interdependent relationships with other professions.

As will be demonstrated throughout this book, the same competencies prove equally fundamental in achieving collaborative person-centred care.

CHALLENGE

- How does the idea of IPE compare to your recent experience of learning?

- If your education didn't include timetabled learning with people from other disciplines, what subject areas do you think you could have studied with others and why?

   ▪ What do you think are the benefits of IPE?

   ▪ Are there any disadvantages to IPE?

The next step

The next phase in the interprofessional education agenda will be the recognition that, as Barr *et al.* (2006) suggest, 'interprofessional education is not an end in itself simply a means of preparing different types of health personnel to work together'. IPE provides a vehicle through which collaborative person-centred practice will be achieved. The recognition that IPE is indeed a means to an end and not an end in itself can be witnessed in the developing Canadian Model (Health Canada 2003), which may prove an important stepping stone in the evolution of collaborative working. Known as the Memorial University Interprofessional Education for Collaborative Person-Centred Practice Initiative, this encourages discussion and debate centring on collaborative *working in practice* – thus discussion focusing on the outcome of the journey as opposed to the vehicle of travel.

The initiative seeks to promote and demonstrate the potential benefits of interprofessional education as a means of achieving collaborative person-centred practice by influencing curriculum designers, thus maximising the number of health professionals 'trained' for person-centred interprofessional team practice and also stimulating networking and sharing of best practice for collaborative person-centred practice. (Herbert 2005) The first phase of the initiative (2003–04) reviewed existing models of interprofessional education and the promotion of collaborative practice, drawing the conclusion that the available published literature to support interprofessional education is thin; a conclusion supported by numerous studies across the UK and US (Zwarenstein *et al.* 2001). However, Herbert (2005) concluded that the absence of evidence of benefit does not necessarily equate to evidence of no benefit, and on that basis further work needed to be commissioned. Phase two (2004–08) seeks to provide the evidence base that will serve to convince faculty members, deans, directors and accrediting bodies that there is a body of knowledge that addresses issues such as how much of a curriculum needs to be common or shared, and how often and in what format this collaborative interaction needs to take place to ensure that health and social care professionals develop the requisite knowledge, attitudes and skills to engage in collaborative person-centred practice (Herbert 2005).

The work of D'Amour and Oandasan (2005) is helpful in moving this debate forward, providing a conceptual framework to describe and link the various elements of interprofessional education and collaborative person-centred practice. (This is one of an excellent series of articles published in the May 2005 supplement to the *Journal of Interprofessional Care*, which includes a full review of the Health Canada Initiative providing an in-depth review of IPE and CPCP.) In brief, D'Amour and Oandasan (*ibid.*) offer a framework linking IPE and CPCP, as illustrated in Figure 1.1.

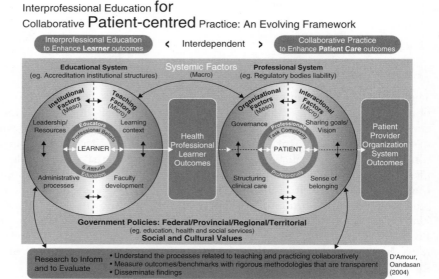

Figure 1.1 Interprofessional education for collaborative patient-centred practice.
Source: D'Amour, D. & Oondasan, I. (2005) Interprofessionality as the field of interprofessional practice and interprofessional education: An emerging concept, *Journal of Interprofessional Care*, May 2005 supplement, 1: 8–20. Reprinted by permission of the publisher (Taylor & Francis Ltd, http://www.informaworld.com).

The D'Amour and Oandasan framework suggests two intimately linked 'circles' of activity: education and practice. The 'education circle' includes factors affecting a health professional learner's capacity to become a competent collaborative practitioner. Importantly, the learner is at the centre and core of the circle and is affected by all factors influencing his or her ability to gain the competencies needed to be able to work collaboratively with other health care professionals. The 'practice circle' comprises processes and factors that affect patient care outcomes in collaborative practice settings. The circle shows the processes through which health professionals structure their collaboration.

D'Amour and Oandasan suggest that the processes that interconnect these circles are both complex and dynamic, concerning human interaction between professionals from different world views within a complex, changing environment. Considering the interaction and interconnectivity between the two circles, they suggest, will assist our understanding of how meeting the needs of clients is critically dependent on the practitioner's ability to work collaboratively. To be effective, person-centred collaborative practice must address the needs of the patients/clients and their wishes; their readiness and willingness to collaborate in their care must be understood. D'Amour and Oandasan (*ibid.*) suggest, 'if we train competent collaborative practitioners, more collaborative practice settings will be developed over time. With increased numbers of settings, more opportunities for learning and teaching collaboration are envisioned. Hence practice is linked with education.'

An alternative, and compelling, perspective on interprofessional education and collaborative practice is provided by Trevillion and Bedford (2003) who suggest, given that there are few uncontested role models of either interprofessional work in practice or interprofessional education, that it is somewhat surprising that IPE has now become the cornerstone of new reforms in social work. They present an intriguing argument that interprofessional education and interprofessional work in practice can usefully be considered as a Wittgensteinian 'language game' within which general concepts are not always a common property of particular instances: a family is a set of overlapping 'likenesses' that cannot be reduced to a single common factor (Wittgenstein 1975: 17). Applying this model to interprofessional practice and the absence of a single defining characteristic of interprofessionalism should not be viewed as an obstacle to meaningful discussion or debate, but rather as an opportunity to explore new avenues of enquiry, thus permitting and facilitating consideration of 'similarity and difference'.

The future

The purpose of this and subsequent chapters is to encourage debate beyond interprofessional education, and to reflect on the next phase of development. Should we be concerned about whether IPE is adopted by all UK health and social care educational institutions or about the actions that educators and practitioners need to take to ensure that the 'implant is not rejected', or should we focus on the journey's destination – collaborative person-centred practice? Milburn and Colyer (2007) suggest that health and social care services will increasingly require practitioners to work more effectively together at the interface of individual professional practice. Achieving effective collaborative interprofessional working will require practitioners to balance their professional, personal and contextualised interprofessional knowledge in a way unique to every interprofessional interaction, driven by the need to achieve person-centred care. IPE cannot teach interprofessional knowledge; rather it should facilitate interprofessional practice, through which such knowledge is construed and person-centred care can be more effectively achieved. Interprofessional practice is highly contextualised by practice setting and point-of-service delivery. Any attempt to decontextualise it for the purpose of curriculum development would be illogical; interprofessional knowledge is in a symbiotic relationship with its prior professional knowledge. IPE should be driven by the natural alliance of complementary professions in order to maximise its potential effectiveness and credibility with practitioners. Recognition of these issues would, in the view of Milburn and Colyer (2007), ensure that IPE initiatives underpin more securely the effective collaboration of professional practitioners in health and social care.

CHALLENGE

The highest-quality professional practice can only be delivered by professionals who are confident and competent and who understand profession-specific practice delivered collaboratively in a person-centred manner, if those professionals endorse the importance of interprofessional practice. To what extent do you agree with this statement?

■ What do your clients want from you as a professional practitioner?

■ How would you define collaborative person-centred care?

■ When and where in the learning cycle of your education should interprofessional learning be positioned to have most benefit to you and ultimately your client group?

■ How can practitioners and teachers ensure that an appropriate balance is achieved between professional and interprofessional knowledge to ensure the delivery of a high-quality, client-focused service?

References

Allsop, J. (1995) *Health Policy and the NHS towards 2000*, 2nd edn. London: Longman.

Baldwin, D. (1996) Some historical notes on interdisciplinary and interprofessional education and practice in healthcare in the USA. *Journal of Interprofessional Care*, 10: 173–87.

Balint, E. (1969) The possibilities of patient-centred medicine. *Journal of the Royal College of General Practitioners*, 17: 269–76.

Barr, H. (1994) NVQs and their implications for interprofessional collaboration. In A. Leathard (ed.), *Going Interprofessional: Working Together for Health and Welfare*. London: Routledge.

Barr, H. (2000) *Cultivating Collaboration Worldwide*. London: CAIPE.

Barr, H (2002) *Interprofessional Education: Today, Yesterday and Tomorrow*. London: LTSN for Health Sciences and Practice.

Barr, H., Freeth, D., Hammick, M., Koppel, I. & Reeves, S. (2006) The evidence base and recommendations for interprofessional education in health and social care. *Journal of Interprofessional Care*, January, 2091: 75–8.

Biggs, S. (1993) User participation and interprofessional collaboration in community care. *Journal of Interprofessional Care*, 7(2): 151–9

Blakemore, K. (2003) *Social Policy: An Introduction*. Buckingham: Open University Press.

Bungay, H. (2001) Pathways in the diagnosis and treatment of breast cancer: The significance of delay. Unpublished PhD thesis, University of Kent at Canterbury.

Bury, M. (1997) *Health and Illness in a Changing Society*. London: Routledge.

Byrne, P. & Long, B. (1976) *Doctors Talking to Patients*. London: HMSO.

Canadian Institute for Health Information (2003) *Health Care in Canada Report*. Canadian Institute for Health Information, http://secure.cihi.ca/cihiweb/dispPage. jsp?cw_page=PG_27_E&cw_topic=27&cw_rel=AR_43_E#full:.

Cleghorn, G.D. & Baker, G.R. (2000) What faculties need to learn about improvement and how to teach it to each other. *Journal of Interprofessional Care*, 14: 147–59.

Colyer, H. & Smith, A. (2008) *Learning and teaching for collaborative practice. Report on the evaluation of the Collaborative Practice module*. Canterbury Christ Church University.

Coulter, A. (2002) After Bristol: Putting patients at the centre, *British Medical Journal*, 342: 648–51.

Counsell, S.R., Kennedy, R.D., Szwabo, P., Wadsworth, N.S. & Wohlgemuth, C. (1999) Curriculum recommendations for residents training in Geriatrics Interdisciplinary Team Care. *Journal of the American Geriatrics Association*, 47: 1145–8.

Crow, J., Smith, L. & Jones, S. (2005) Using the patchwork text as a vehicle for promoting interprofessional health and social care collaboration in higher education. *Learning in Health and Social Care*, 4(3): 117–28.

Curran, V. (2004) *Interprofessional Education for Collaborative Patient-Centred Practice*. Research synthesis paper, http://www.hc-sc.gc.ca/hsc-sss/hhr-rhs/strateg/interprof/synth_e.html.

D'Amour, D. & Oandasan, I. (2005) Interprofessionality as the field of interprofessional practice and interprofessional education: An emerging concept. *Journal of Interprofessional Care*, May, Supplement, 1: 8–20.

Dalton, S., Spencer, J., Dunn, M., Albert, E, Walker, J. & Farrell, G. (2003) Re-thinking approaches to undergraduate health professional education: Interdisciplinary rural placement programme. *Collegian*, 10(1): 17–21.

Department of Health (1991) *The Patient's Charter*. London: HMSO.

Department of Health (2000) *The NHS Plan*. London: Department of Health.

Department of Health (2001a) *National Service Framework for Older People*. London: Department of Health.

Department of Health (2001b) *Valuing People: A New Strategy for Learning Disability in the 21st Century*. London: Department of Health.

Department of Health (2001c) *Shifting the Balance of Power within the NHS: Securing Delivery*. London: Department of Health.

Department of Health (2001d) *The Expert Patient: A New Approach to Chronic Disease Management in the 21st Century*. London: Department of Health.

Department of Health (2007a) *Our NHS, Our Future: NHS Next Stage Review – Interim Report*. London: Department of Health.

Department of Health (2007b) *What Matters to our Patients, Public and Staff*. London, Department of Health.

Dewing, J. (2004) Concerns relating to the application of frameworks to promote person-centredness in nursing with older people. *International Journal of Older People Nursing*, 13(3a): 39–44.

Dowling, S., Manthorpe, J. & Cowley, S. (2006), *Person-Centred Planning in Social Care*. http://www.jrf.org.uk/bookshop/eBooks/9781859354803.pdf, accessed November 2007.

Gelmon, S., White, A., Carlson, L. & Norman, L. (2000) Making organizational change to achieve improvement and interprofessional learning: Perspectives from health professions educators. *Journal of Interprofessional Care*, 14: 131–46.

Hall, P. (2005) Interprofessional teamwork: Professional cultures as barriers. *Journal of Interprofessional Care*, May, Supplement, 1: 188–96.

Ham, C. (1992) *Health Policy in Britain*, 3rd edn. Macmillan: Basingstoke.

Health Canada (2003) *First Ministers' Accord on Healthcare Renewal*. Ottawa: Health Canada.

Herbert, C. (2005) Changing the culture: Interprofessional education for collaborative patient-centred pratice in Canada. *Journal of Interprofessional Care*, May, Supplement, 1: 1–4.

Humphris, D. & Clark, J. (2007) Embedding interprofessional learning in Hampshire and the Isle of Wight: The New Generation Project in piloting interprofessional education: Four English case studies. Occasional Paper No. 8, July. York: Higher Education Academy.

Improving Outcomes in Breast Cancer (1996) *Guidance for Purchasers. The Research Evidence*. Cancer Guidance Sub-group of the Clinical Outcomes Group, NHS Executive, London: Department of Health.

Kennedy, I. (2001) *Learning from Bristol: The Report of the Public Inquiry into Children's Heart Surgery at the Bristol Royal Infirmary 1984–1995*. Command Paper CM 5207. London: HMSO.

Knapp, M., Bennett, N., Plumb, J. & Robinson, J. (2000) Community-based quality improvement education for health professions: Balancing benefits for communities and students. *Journal of Interprofessional Care*, 14: 119–30.

Leathard, A. (1994) Interprofessional developments in Britain: An overview. In A. Leathard (ed.), *Going Interprofessional: Working Together for Health and Welfare*. London: Routledge.

McWhinney, I. (1989) The need for a transformed clinical method. In M. Stewart & D. Roter (eds), *Communicating with Medical Patients*. London: Sage.

Mead, N. & Bower, P. (2000) Patient centredness: A conceptual framework and review of the empirical literature. *Social Science and Medicine*, 51: 1087–110.

Milburn, P. & Colyer, H. (2007) Professional knowledge and interprofessional practice. *Radiography*, Oct., in press, doi:10.1016/j.radi.2007.09.003.

Neuberger, J. & Tallis, R. (1999) Do we need a new word for patients? *British Medical Journal*, 318: 1756–8.

O'Halloran, C., Hean, S., Humphris, D. & Macleod-Clark, J. (2006) Developing common learning: The New Generation Project undergraduate curriculum model. *Journal of Interprofessional Care*, January, 20(1): 12–28.

Parsell, G. & Bligh, J. (1998) Interprofessional learning. *Postgraduate Medical Journal*, 74(868): 89–95.

Payne, M. (1997) *Social Work Theory*, 2nd edn. Basingstoke: Palgrave Macmillan.

Pollard, K., Sellman, D. & Senior, B. (2005) The need for interprofessional working. In Barrett, G., Sellman, D. & Thomas, J. (eds) *Interprofessional Working in Health and Social Care: Professional Perspectives*. Basingstoke: Palgrave Macmillan.

Price, B. (2006) Exploring person-centred care. *Nursing Standard*, 20(50): 49–56.

Reeves, S. (2000) Community-based interprofessional education for medical, nursing and dental students. *Health and Social Care in the Community*, 8(4): 269–76.

Reeves, S. (2001) A systematic review of the effects of interprofessional education on staff involved in the care of adults with mental health problems. *Journal of Psychiatric and Mental Health Nursing*, 8: 533–42.

Royal College of Nursing (2004) *Interprofessional Education – A Literature Review*. London: Royal College of Nursing.

Szasz, G. (1969) Interprofessional education in the health sciences. *Millbank Memorial Fund Quarterly*, 47: 449–75.

Trevillion, S. & Bedford, L. (2003) Utopianism and the pragmatism in interprofessional education. *Social Work Education*, 22(2): 215–27.

Wilcock, P. & Headrick, L. (2000) Interprofessional learning for the improvement of health care: Why bother? *Journal of Interprofessional Care*, 14(2): 11–17

Wittengenstein, L. (1975) *The Blue and Brown Book: Preliminary Studies for the Philosophical Investigations*. Oxford. Blackwell.

Witz, A (1992) *Professions and Patriarchy*. Routledge: London.

World Health Organisation (1987) *Learning Together to Work Together for Health. Report of a WHO Study Group on Multiprofessional Education of Health Personnel: The Team Approach*. Technical report series 768. Geneva: World Health Organisation.

Zwarenstein, M., Reeves, S., Barr, H., Hammick, M., Koppel, I. & Atkins, J. (2001) Interprofessional education: Effects on professional practice and health care outcomes. *Cochrane Database of Systematic Reviews* 91: CD002213. Oxford: Cochrane Library.

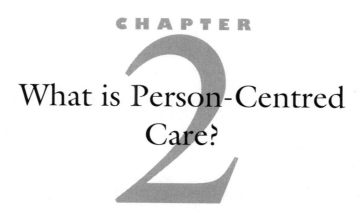

CHAPTER 2

What is Person-Centred Care?

Paul Elliott and Georgina Koubel

Person-centred care is a key theme for health and social care and is central to the ways in which health and social care practitioners engage with the people who use services. In interprofessional working it is particularly important to be aware of the potential for professional organisations, discourses and perspectives to overwhelm the individuals (and their families/carers) whose views, interests and choices should be at the centre of intervention by health and social care services. However, before we look at the ways in which person-centred care informs practice, it is important to address the concept itself. This chapter therefore aims to:

- Develop your understanding of the concept of person-centred care.

- Explore the origins of person-centred care in relation to interprofessional working in the current climate of health and social care.

- Facilitate your knowledge and application of the theoretical and value frameworks that inform person-centred care.

- Develop your ability to reflect on the concept of person-centred care and the importance of adopting a holistic, non-discriminatory and biopsychosocial as opposed to biomedical approach (Ogden 2007).

- Analyse the way in which person-centred care relates to good practice with individuals who use health and social care services.

In writing this chapter our intention is to introduce you to the idea of person-centred care as a concept that should always underpin health and social care practice. In doing this we will reflect on the historical basis of person-centred care, followed by reflection on what person-centred care is. The chapter also focuses on a number of theoretical frameworks that inform person-centred care. Engagement with health and social care systems inevitably reflects the ways in which society constructs the relationships between professionals and service users. At times person-centred care challenges the norms and attitudes of society, particularly in relation to people who may be seen as vulnerable or marginalised. Because of their particular attention to excluded or vulnerable groups, we also look at the development of social work values and how these relate to the construction and application of person-centred care.

We will introduce you to a range of theoretical perspectives that can serve to promote or hinder the successful application of person-centred care. In addition, in analysing a number of factors that militate against the application of person-centred approaches, we offer discussion related to the importance of challenging the status quo as a means of ensuring that the frontiers of person-centred care are always moving forward. Throughout the chapter we present a series of reflective exercises and challenges aimed at generating critical think-ing and analysis.

A brief history of person-centred perspectives

In appreciating the importance of adopting a person-centred approach to health or social care practice, we need to consider the historical perspective. Where does the concept of person-centred care originate? What is person-cen-tred care?

Although there is no specific literature to identify the origins of person-cen-tred care, the concepts that underpin the idea can be found within the biblical context, within the context of human rights, health and safety law and psychol-ogy, and within the professional codes of conduct of the health and social care professions. From a biblical perspective, the church provided a basic support network for those who were unable to care for themselves. Such support can be traced back to the Crusades where the Knights Templar order was founded to protect travellers moving through the Holy Land towards Jerusalem from marauding bands of robbers. Its actions were both supported and rewarded by the Pope of the time (Martin 2004).

During the reign of Elizabeth I, circa 1601, the Poor Laws were intro-duced in an attempt to address the needs of the sick and infirm (Bloy 2002). Furthermore, the concept of person-centred care can be linked to what Smith (1998) outlines as circuits of knowledge. These can be adapted to reflect four distinct circuits:

■ The *theological circuit* centred on beliefs about the person and human need that are espoused by the church, faith and divinity. Within this understanding of person-centred care, the church can be identified as the principal provider of care for individuals, and obedience to the teachings of the church would facilitate this. In this circuit, knowledge of what being 'person centred' meant was dictated by theological interpretation. In other words, society was God centred and in the Judeo-Christian value system that then informed Western thinking around helping those who were sick or disadvantaged, God could be served by considering and tending to the needs of others.

■ The *scientific circuit* centres beliefs about the person and human need on the notion of objective fact involving the scientific method, reason, objective truth and a biomedical approach (Ogden 2007). The Enlightenment emerged from the strong, almost exclusive focus on religious values that characterised mediaeval society. Science, logic, deduction and reason were its watchwords. This was to suggest that if something could not be proved rationally or empirically, it held no validity. In this perspective, being person centred is perceived to be underpinned by factual knowledge, as opposed to subjective belief as was the case within the theological circuit. Therefore within a scientific context, to be person centred was about being clinically objective as opposed to acknowledging such feelings as partiality, compassion, kindness, empathy or benevolence. This largely informed the scientific development of medical science.

■ The *humanistic circuit* centres on beliefs about the person relating to concepts of individuality, human rights and a biopsychosocial or holistic approach (Engle 1980). This circuit has a good deal in common with current thinking about what person-centred care should be. This values the importance of recognising the individuality of each and every person, the right of each individual to be treated with understanding, dignity and equality, and the recognition that person-centred care must involve acknowledging the physical, psychological and social needs of each individual. This links back to the teachings of Judeo-Christian philosophy and the notions of Kantian philosophy, whereby every individual is seen as a person of value in their own right rather than as a possible means to an end (Singer 1994), even where that 'end' may be of benefit to humanity in general. This perspective informs many of the ethical debates of our times, such as those relating to cloning and the generation of stem cells to deal with disease and impairment.

■ The *social circuit* represents an alternative way of thinking about humanity taking a social or sociological perspective. This sets the individual in the context of their social groupings such as 'class', 'race', 'gender', 'age', '(dis)ability' and 'sexuality' and looks at the constructs and assumptions that can be attributed to people as a result of these. The social model also encompasses notions of citizenship, rights and social justice, whereby people are seen in their political context as well as within the traditional person-centred values of social work and social care.

================= **CHALLENGE** =================

■ What do you think about these different perspectives?

■ Do you recognise your own way of thinking within one or other of these circuits?

- How do they affect your approach to life generally?

- Can you think how they would affect your practice?

The notion that individuals should be entitled to information and support has served to inform the conceptual development of person-centred care as we know it today and these principles are set out within the codes of conduct produced by a range of professional bodies and legislation, such as international health and safety laws (Taylor 2002) and the principles underpinning human rights. Within the context of human rights, person-centred care is about the protection of life, the prohibition of torture, freedom of thought and conscience and freedom of expression (Wilkinson & Caulfield 2001).

The professionals who work in the fields of health and social care are fundamentally influenced by their professional education and status to see themselves as providers of services that should be (more or less) gratefully received by those who are subject to them. Professionals are expected to have a duty of care and work for the best interests of the people who use services. Laws, policies and codes of conduct encompass, enable and curtail professional activities and interactions with individuals who use services. Government recognition that certain groups, such as those with learning disabilities, have been particularly marginalised and discriminated against throughout history has given rise to specific policies, such as person-centred planning, based on the White Paper *Valuing Difference* (Department of Health 2001).

Professional ethical codes stress the need for professionals to be accountable for their practice and for the rights of service users to autonomy within the decision-making process and to have their views and preferences respected, assuming an appropriate level of capacity to make those choices and understand the consequences of their decisions (Koubel 2006). This indicates that the application of person-centred care should reflect a partnership between professionals and the individual seeking health or social care intervention. However, there are a number of reasons this is not always the case. One of the many ways in which professionals can unwittingly disempower and discriminate against the people who seek their interventions is in their use of language. Any use of scientific language or professional jargon in conversations with individuals that is unfamiliar to people outside the profession is alienating and inhibits their ability to play a full role in discussions around their problems or the solutions that may be appropriate in their resolution (Thompson 2007).

CHALLENGE

- How can professionals use their power to promote partnership working rather than undermine it?

- Can you identify any occasions where you have been aware of where professional language could make it more difficult to promote person-centred care?

Empowerment

The concept of empowerment and the way in which power is unde within the relations between individuals seeking health and social care in vention and health and social care practitioners is so important that we need to think a bit about it before moving on. Power is a difficult concept to define. In itself it is neither good nor bad, but is rather dependent on how it used and by whom, to what end and how it reflects social relations.

Certain groups in society may be seen as being particularly vulnerable and powerless, such as the very young or the very old, people with mental health problems or disabilities, or those who are excluded from mainstream society because of homelessness, offending behaviour or cultural and ethnic differences. However, this does not mean that such people are completely powerless or that the issues that increase their vulnerability cannot be challenged. Thompson (2005) addresses this simplistic or reductionist concept of power and proposes an integrated model that is useful to health and social care professionals in helping us to understand the complex way in which power works. He calls this the PCS model, which recognises that people may be disempowered through:

- *Personal or psychological problems or prejudices*, which may be reinforced by the attitudes and expectations of others. These may be seen in relation to the personal or psychological attributes of those seeking health or social care intervention, but may equally relate to those professionals who work in the services. This will be addressed later in the chapter.

- *Cultural factors* such as the discourses around, which may lead to discrimination against, for example, older or disabled people if it is assumed that they are inevitably less able and should be protected from taking risks or making decisions in same ways as other people. This is frequently found within the inter-professional discourse. Conflicts arising among professionals may often be reflected in taken-for-granted attitudes and assumptions that are not shared by different disciplines or group members.

- *Structural issues*, which depend on the way in which society is structured to favour, for example, white middle-class heterosexual men and discriminates against or oppresses people like asylum seekers, people who are living with HIV/Aids or those who do not contribute to the 'production' of goods in society (older people, those on benefits) and who may then be construed as a 'burden' on society.

Awareness of our own personal prejudices, alongside knowledge of the significance of cultural stereotypes and the impact of social disadvantage, can be helpful in recognising the potential for the power of professionals and organisations to disadvantage or disempower those seeking health or social care intervention. It is therefore an extremely useful model in helping us to understand some of the complexities of person-centred care. The concept of stereotyping and awareness of our own personal prejudices is developed further in Chapter 4.

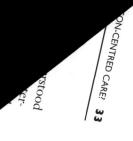

===== **CHALLENGE** =====

help you to think about person-centred care?

question some of the images and ideas that society produces in
disempowers or marginalises?

ys in which this would be reflected in the attitudes and practice

Communication

Before we look further at empowerment in relation to person-centred care, it is important to look at some of the constructs that inform the ways in which we work, and to question some of the ways we think about our work. All interventions we have with others depend on our understanding and skills in communication.

Communication can be broken down into verbal, non-verbal and written. For those involved in the provision of health and social care, all of these elements are essential to ensuring that interventions are person centred. For example, where verbal communication is concerned it is not simply what we say or how we may say it. It is also about the context in which we say it, the tone of voice in which we speak and the accent we have. Where people have specific communication needs such as hearing difficulties or a different language, it is essential for practitioners to consider how these can be accommodated to ensure that the person is involved in the communication.

Non-verbal communication may be about the gestures we make, our facial expressions, the stance we take, our proximity to an individual we are interacting with and how we are dressed. Non-verbal communication can convey a great deal about the respect we have towards an individual, about how welcome their views are and whether we are attentive to their needs and wishes.

Written communication is about the script we use, the legibility of our writing, the location where the written word appears and semantics used. For example, and from personal experience of reading clinical notes: *bitten by dog, terrified of rabies, dog OK!* All of these elements can affect the quality of the person-centred care provided.

Those involved in the provision of health and social care must continually be aware of the ways in which we apply all three forms of communication. Applied wrongly, they can have a significant impact on the degree to which others perceive how person centred the interventions were. Professionals also need to be aware that the Data Protection Act (1998) gives individuals the right to see the records kept about them.

===== **CHALLENGE** =====

- Regarding each form of communication, can you think of examples where your interventions may have been perceived as positive or negative?

■ In thinking about what you write about people, how is this changed by knowing they have the right to see it for themselves?

■ What would you not want them to see?

■ What would you not want to see written about you or someone dear to you?

■ How could this affect the effectiveness of written communication?

As professionals, we have to be continually aware of the impact of our communication and our use of language, both when working with individuals and when discussing them with other members of the interprofessional team. The words we use and the way we use them convey very clearly our values and attitudes towards others. Terms that were acceptable at one time may change. This is more than 'political correctness'. The use of such terms may cause emotional and social harm and result in the generation of preconceived perceptions of individuals. Such preconceived perceptions are not consistent with the philosophy of person-centred care.

Awareness of the possible pejorative connotations of the words that professionals apply to those who use services is an important feature in understanding the potential for practice to be discriminatory and disempowering. (The issue of communication is explored further by Barber, McLaughlin and Wood in Chapter 4.) The values underpinning all professional disciplines (codes of conduct) specifically address this power imbalance between the professional worker and others, and highlight the need for a move away from 'a paternalistic "looking after these poor people" approach towards a genuine aim of empowerment and maximum independence' (Thompson 2005: 148; Neuberger & Tallis 1999). A brief consideration of the connections between person-centred care and professional values will be useful in trying to help us get to the root of the meaning and application of person-centred care.

Professional values and their application to person-centred care

All health and social work is ultimately about people, so how can the idea of person-centred care be problematic? What room could there be for tensions and conflicts? Where are these likely to occur for health and social care professionals within the interprofessional context?

One of the key factors in the development of professional values in the 1950s and 1960s was the determination to avoid any possible repetition of the atrocious scenes witnessed (and sometimes, shockingly, administered) by health and social care workers in Germany during the Second World War (Lorenz 1994). Following the person-centred therapeutic model (Rogers 1961), in 1969 Biestek (a former monk) identified a number of principles that he held should inform therapeutic practice (Moss 2007). Despite the changes in the environment in which health and social care are practised today and the

language in which his ideas are expressed, Biestek's seven key principles reso-
nate closely with the concept of person-centred care (*ibid.*). These are:

- Individualisation.

- Purposeful expression of feelings.

- Controlled emotional involvement.

- Acceptance.

- Non-judgemental attitude.

- Client self-determination.

- Confidentiality.

━━━━━━━━━━━━━━━━━━━━━━━━ **CHALLENGE** ━━━━━━━━━━━━━━━━━━━━━━━━

Look at each of the above principles and think carefully about what they really mean.

- Think about the possible difficulties you would encounter as a practitioner in trying to
  adhere to each of them.

- Discuss what you could do to address these conflicts.

- Can you think of other principles that would help you to carry out your role more
  effectively?

The social model that emerged following this period was based on the principles of universality and collectivity, where people paid into a system when
they were working and were entitled to benefits in times of sickness or unem-
ployment. Responding to concerns about the effectiveness of such social interventions and the cost of the welfare state, alongside ideological changes in
revisiting the role of the state in relation to health and welfare, the welfare
agenda became increasingly dominated by competing rights, responsibilities
and resources. The National Health Service (NHS) and Community Care Act
(1990) changed the argument away from the realities of being poor and disadvantaged to focus on the consumerisation of the relationship between health
and social care professionals and those seeking their intervention (Dominelli
2004).

Brown (2004: 17) provides a useful synopsis of the changes that are happening in the context of health and welfare services:

> The focus on the undeniable changes in the welfare services, and how they are
> organised, managed and delivered, diverts attention from the unchanging reali-
> ties of being poor, being alone, experiencing health problems, becoming older
> and living in a society which discriminates against people who are different,
> whether through class, gender, age, ethnicity, disability sexuality or any other
> social division.

Person-centred care can therefore be seen as having relevance to social values, both the political dimension that focuses on issues of citizen's rights and social justice, and the interpersonal imperatives of respecting and meeting the needs of individuals and their families or carers. This is not to say that all people's needs and rights can be met by health and social care services, or that there are no conflicts. For example, health and social care professionals have to manage tensions between the needs of children and their parents' rights to respect for their family life.

A further dilemma exists where the wishes of the family or friends of the individual conflict with the wishes and preferences of the individual seeking or receiving intervention. In situations where the service user may be frail, forgetful or where their voice is minimised by communication difficulties or marginalised by inexperience of having a choice or lack of opportunities to build communication skills, it is extremely easy for other people to think they know what is best for that person (Shakespeare 2000).

Empowerment, independence and choice are not easy concepts and have complex meanings and implications for practice. Although they are generally understood as crucial to the role of health and social care workers in relation to those seeking their intervention in the struggle not to foster dependence or abuse of professional power, it is not always clear how these ideas translate into practice. Take for an example the misuse of personal power within an infection-prevention context: 'I do not have time to wash my hands. I am too busy meeting the needs of those I am providing care for' (Elliott 2003a).

Driven by the concepts of rights, choices and seeing individuals who use services as experts in their own condition by virtue of their experiences may be challenging to those who were previously perceived as the experts; that is, doctors, nurses, other allied health professionals and social workers. Despite the many years over which professionals may have studied and the experience they may have gained in professional practice, the experience of those living with a condition is bound to have been different.

CHALLENGE

Consider the following:

- When patients, clients or service users disagree with the multiprofessional team, what is the role of the professional?

- Where do your sympathies, interests and loyalties lie?

- What if you disagree with the team?

- Is it your role to be the person's advocate?

- What are the personal, professional and organisational dilemmas facing you in such situations?

- How does such a situation relate to the notion of person-centred care?

While the notion of empowerment is a key feature of professional practice, it inevitably entails potential clashes with the equally important area around assessing and managing risk. In this context, risk may involve the individual seeking health or social care intervention, their carers or families, the general public and the professional. The balance between acceptable levels of risk, dangers to oneself or others and the freedom of the individual is not always an easy area for practitioners to struggle with. The choices exercised by an individual may be unwise and even unsafe. The question for professionals is how person-centred practice can address these issues without compromising the autonomy of the individual.

Even where the person concerned is used to expressing themselves and clear about what their needs are, it can be difficult for professionals to think of the person as an expert in their own condition. For example, the disability movement in the UK aims far beyond the push for better services and more consultation with people with disabilities towards a reconstruction of the notion of disability itself. Taking the social model of disability as its foundation (Southampton Centre for Independent Living, n.d.), it focuses not on the limitations caused by the impairment of the individual, but on the barriers existing in society to full participation by people with disabilities. Disability and dependence are notions that have a long history and changing the balance of power in relation to disability, specifically by people who themselves experience disabilities, remains a challenge (Swain *et al.* 2005).

Thompson (2007) equates the discrimination that disabled people face with the kinds of discrimination and prejudice existing towards people of a different race, class or gender. In addition to the problems posed by the attitudes of individuals (who may be in a position of power through their roles as employers, professionals and so on), there is a process of systemic discrimination that constructs as inherently dependent the person with disabilities or older person, and infantilises them as incapable and unequal.

Other models that inform person-centred care

All professionals are committed in theory to the idea that the individual person is the centre of their intervention. There is a temptation to think about person-centred care as something that is inimical to health and social care. However, this is clearly not always the case. This part of the chapter will therefore look more closely at the factors, both psychological and institutional, that can get in the way of person-centred care even where the professional understands the concept and is motivated to apply it.

Health and safety

From a health and safety perspective, person-centred care is about protecting the welfare of those within the working environment. For the health or social care professional the term *working environment* applies to wherever you are undertaking your professional activities. As Taylor (2002) indicates, health and safety is a global issue and as such, places the concept of person-centred care on a global footing. In effect, everything that a health or social care professional does has implications for person-centred care with regard to promoting the welfare of those seeking their intervention.

For example, the provision of information can serve to link the concept of person-centred care and protecting the health and safety of those seeking our interventions. Individuals have an absolute right to know what they might expect from contact with health and social care professionals and service providers. For example, there have been numerous examples where the health and safety of individuals has been placed at serious risk as a result of information being withheld or taking an extensive period of time to be published. Examination of the UK's Healthcare Commission (2007), Health Protection Agency (2007) and the US Centres for Disease Control and Prevention (2007) websites clearly indicates this where the transmission of methicillin resistant Staphylococcus aureus (MRSA) and Clostridium difficile (C. diff) is concerned.

The concepts that underpin person-centred care can also be linked with a variety of theories and approaches within psychology. Although we provide examples and explanations for each of the theories and approaches outlined, it is important to recognise that none of them exists in isolation. They will all have an impact on person-centred care both individually and together, and influence the way in which health and social care professionals think about the notion of person-centred care and its application to interprofessional practice.

Cognitive dissonance

Festinger (1962) proposes that individuals will attempt to justify what they have done or what they wish to do. As professionals, we must all be aware that person-centred care is not only about informing but explaining and encouraging questioning. Cognitive dissonance is when one behaves in a way that conflicts with one's beliefs. If, for example, a health or social care professional informs an individual of something but then fails to explain the information they have given or does not allow the individual to ask questions, they recognise that this is wrong but attempt to justify it through generating a rationalised excuse. However, such rationalised excuses are not rational. For example, 'I cannot remember everything and anyway they could have asked.' Is this a reasonable approach? Could it be called person centred? Clearly, this constitutes an excuse that is not consistent with person-centred care, but will be likely to make perfect sense to the given professional and psychologically serve to excuse them from responsibility for their failure. Such excuses are in fact a form of defence, in that if these rationalisations were not generated the professional would experience stress as a result of the emotional conflict that would exist between *knowing what they should have done* and *what they actually did*. These rationalisations can have a major impact on the quality of the person-centred care they provide. As such, cognitive dissonance can have a significant impact on an individual's ability to practise in a person-centred way.

================================ **CHALLENGE** ================================

■ Can you think of occasions where you may have made such excuses to justify your practice?

■ How rational do you think your excuse was and what impact did it have on the quality of person-centred care you provided?

In undertaking this reflection exercise and those that follow, you may find it helpful to use the following reflective template (from Elliott 2006):

Reflective point	**Guiding statement**
Who	Who do you think person-centred care applies to?
What	What do you feel person-centred care is about?
When	When is person-centred care necessary?
Where	Where can person-centred care be applied?
How	How have you undertaken person-centred care in the past?
Why	Why is person-centred care necessary?

All of the above points are intended to facilitate your own reflections. However, the final point below is intended to take your thinking beyond that of a subjective perspective. It is asking you to review what you have decided regarding the above six points and challenge your own assumptions.

Who says so	How do I know what I believe and feel is correct ?
	What evidence do I have other than my own perspective to support what I believe and feel?
	Posed with the same situation or event, could another individual have reached the same conclusions as you did?

Locus of control

The concept of health locus of control (Wallston & Wallston 1982) has two dimensions, *internal* and *external*. The former identifies that people who are seeking health or social care intervention should be perceived as equal partners with regard to their health and welfare. Health and social care professionals should actively seek to involve individuals and provide them with appropriate information, and to seek their thoughts and feelings related to the interventions to which they will be subject. For example, as discussed previously, the completion of documentation relevant to an individual's health or social care would involve working with the individual in not only determining what should be written but also the language used, which should be clearly non-discriminatory and without the use of jargon. Within this context, the application of an internal locus of control is consistent with the philosophy of person-centred care. In contrast, an external locus of control is indicative of the health or social carer exerting power and authority over an individual. It is also consistent with egocentrism where, for example, the carer makes the assumption that they know more than the individual about their health or social care problem.

The application of an external locus of control is also indicative of dictating to and directing an individual. For example, within the context of health promotion, the professional may tell an individual that they must give up smoking. Telling someone that they must do something is unlikely to have any consistent effect and is rarely successful, as indicated in the work of Reason *et al.* (1998), Lawton and Parker (1999, 2002) and Parker and Lawton (2003). As such, the application of an external locus of control is not consistent with the philosophy of person-centred care.

=========================== **CHALLENGE** ===========================

■ Take some time to reflect on your own practice and identify situations where you may have adopted both internal and external locus of control approaches.

■ Which had greater success, which were more professional and ethical?

■ Consider in the case of one internal and one external approach the difference in the individual's response to you.

Cognitive economy

Cognitive economy (Roth & Frisby 1992) is a process that is closely linked to cognitive dissonance and as such, can serve to inhibit the application of person-centred care. Within the context of the latter, Reason (1998) identifies that humans continually strive to achieve maximum gain for the minimum amount of thinking. For example, person-centred care may be compromised when a health or social care professional becomes fixated on completing their workload within a specified time period at the expense of others' needs. Such needs might include wishing to ask questions or question something to do with a decision a health or social care professional has made on their behalf. In such a situation, because of the health or social carer's cognitively economic fixation on completing their workload, they will have an increased propensity to dismiss such needs. Clearly, such dismissal is not consistent with person-centred care and may have an impact on an individual's future beliefs about that particular health or social care professional and others members of their given profession.

=========================== **CHALLENGE** ===========================

■ Have there ever been occasions when you may have felt under pressure to complete your workload and as a result, on reflection, feel that you may have dismissed an individual's needs?

■ How person centred do you feel such dismissal is? What else could you have done?

Unrealistic optimism

Unrealistic optimism (Weinstein 1984), within the context of person-centred care, is where a health or social care professional becomes egocentric or overconfident about the degree to which they are practising in a person-centred way. For example, a practitioner may, as a result of being cognitively economic in their thinking, believe that the interventions they make are person centred when in fact they are not. Such a belief can be reinforced by egocentric attitudes, such as 'I am an experienced professional and therefore I would know if my interventions were not person centred'.

However, such attitudes are unrealistic because they are based on the subjective assumption that experience and being person centred are synonymous. Furthermore, such an attitude is optimistic because it is rationalised (dissonanced based), as it provides the professional with a reason to justify that they are person centred in what they do. Such unrealistically optimistic beliefs and attitudes can inhibit the application of person-centred care.

CHALLENGE

- Can you think of an occasion when you have felt that an intervention you made was person centred, but when you now reflect back feel that the intervention was in fact unrealistically optimistic?

Stereotyping

Stereotyping is something that most of us are good at. It allows practitioners to make sense of the setting they practise within, the individuals they interact with and the social context within which they exist. For example:

- The categorisation of an individual by their health problem: 'the appendix in bed 6' or 'the leg ulcer at number 63'.

- Someone being labelled as aggressive because they have a history of mental health problems.

- Making the assumption that living on a council estate indicates that a person is of working class and/or of low intelligence.

- Assuming that because someone comes from a particular ethnic or cultural background, their family will take on their care after discharge.

Each of these examples is consistent with dissonance-based and cognitively economic thinking and may well give rise to interventions or decision frames that do not reflect a person-centred approach, resulting from the generation of preconceived ideas and expectations. For example, have you overheard derogatory or overgeneralised remarks being made about a particular individual? Such an experience may well have caused you to generate an impression about the individual, which may, in turn and without you realising it, have affected the quality of your work in relation to decisions concerning that individual. The concept of stereotyping is discussed further in Chapter 4.

== **CHALLENGE** ==

■ Have there ever been occasions when you have stereotyped individuals according to their age, ethnic background, gender, place of residence, frequency of attendance to see you, health problem or appearance?

■ How might this have affected the degree to which your interaction with an individual was person centred?

These are specific examples of how theory can be translated into practice and affect the provision of person-centred care. However, our ability to be person centred can also be affected by resources, which are human, financial and material constraints. For example, the quality of person-centred care can be directly affected by the amount of money available to supply equipment and employ staff. Time is also a key resource in listening attentively to the needs of an individual, rather than finding a quick and easy (but not necessarily the most effective or preferred) solution that will set the professional free to deal with the next person on the list. If there are insufficient resources, then arguably the potential for quality person-centred care to occur will be reduced. Increased workloads lead to elevated levels of stress and raised sickness rates. This will have a direct impact on the quality of person-centred care provided.

For most of us, health or social care decisions are never easy and at times can be very emotive. In some cases the best we can hope for is to end our working period feeling that we have given the best we can with what we have at our disposal. There is an almost unquestioned assumption that health and social care values and the interventions we make are more or less synonymous with being person centred. Yet that is not necessarily the reality. Many within health and social care purport to provide interventions that are person centred. However, much of what we do is more consistent with a task orientation, getting the job done irrespective of the impact it has on others. Health and social care practice is physically and psychologically demanding. Such demands can place all of us under significant amounts of stress, which in turn can result in high levels of fatigue, sickness and low morale. Subsequently, the propensity for a health or social care professional to become task oriented as opposed person centred is very high.

== **CHALLENGE** ==

Take some time to think about whether your practice is really person centred or task oriented. In doing this you might want to take into account the following:

■ How much stress am I under within my professional practice/student role?

■ What is the state of my morale?

■ How well am I supported in my role and the decisions I have to take?

■ To what extent do these factors affect my ability and desire to be person centred?

Having undertaken the challenge above, you may feel that being person centred can not only be difficult at times but also can very much depend on how we feel. How we feel affects how we think (Elliott 2003b) and how we perceive both our own professional practice and the professional practice of others. For example, imagine you are observing a colleague's practice. From your observations you will draw intuitive conclusions about the professionalism and quality of what your colleague is doing. However, your conclusions are based on what you subjectively believe being professional is and what constitutes quality practice to be. Yet how do you know that the conclusions you have drawn are a true representation of what was actually happening? What is person centred to you may not be the same for another person. Each of us has our own idea of what constitutes person-centred care and arguably, such differences in interpretation can in themselves result in practice not being person centred. Furthermore, if your perception of what constitutes person-centred care is not consistent with what your colleague believes, that may result in you stereotyping your colleague in a negative way. Such negative stereotyping is in itself not consistent with a person-centred approach.

═══════════════════ **CHALLENGE** ═══════════════════

■ Have there ever been occasions when your beliefs about person-centred care have not been consistent with a colleague's and as a result of this you have had a difference of opinion?

■ Did this alter your thinking about your colleague's practice?

■ What did you do/could you have done to challenge their practice?

Thus far we have considered person-centred care within the context of making actual interventions. Yet sometimes being person centred is about doing nothing at all. For example, an underpinning philosophy of health and social care from the point at which we first encounter an individual seeking our intervention is their eventual discharge. As such, there will be occasions when we have to stand back and encourage/allow individual to achieve goals for themselves. However, on occasions this may be interpreted by the individual and their family or friends as not being consistent with a person-centred approach. In reality, facilitating an individual to achieve their own goals is absolutely consistent with being person centred, but the individual, their family and friends may need this to be explained to them.

The whole point of being person centred is to move beyond dissonance-based, cognitively economic and unrealistically optimistic perspectives towards adopting a more holistic view, where each individual's needs are considered in the light of their particular health or social care-related problems.

Having considered the issues and theories that inform person-centred care, you may be wondering how all this relates to the actual practice of health and social care. Take a look at the following case study and think carefully about the relevance for your own perspective and the relationship between the concepts of partnership, person-centred care and inter-professional practice.

CASE STUDY: THE CHALLENGE OF REMAINING PERSON CENTRED IN PRACTICE

Anna Rashid is a 47-year-old academic researcher who has been badly injured following a car crash that broke her spine. Unable to use her legs and with limited movement in her arms, Anna has been told that she will have to relearn most of the activities of daily living (Roper *et al.* 2000). At present Anna is in hospital, but she is now well enough to be considered for discharge. She has two children aged 7 and 12 who are currently being cared for by her parents. Her house is being adapted to accommodate a wheelchair and Anna is being offered daily physiotherapy to build up the muscles that she can use to encourage her independence, but she is clearly not motivated to take advantage of this.

The consultant has suggested that Anna should go into a care home or rehabilitation centre for six months so that she can continue to progress towards managing her own personal care. However, Anna is becoming depressed in hospital. She says that she wants to go home, look after her children and get back to work. The professionals involved believe this is unrealistic, as Anna becomes quite exhausted and depressed following her physiotherapy sessions, which only last an hour.

CHALLENGE

Before you read on, think about the following issues:

■ As a person, how do you think you would want to be treated in this sort of situation?

■ As a member of the interprofessional team, how would you address this conflict?

■ How can you approach this situation in a way that recognises Anna's rights as a person and promotes her independence as fully as possible?

CASE STUDY continued

One way of achieving these aims would be to draw up a plan for Anna that would do the following:

■ Provide a chart that identifies the progress Anna is making step by step, on a daily basis, thereby enhancing her sense of achievement.

■ Do this over an extended period, with a realistic date being set for when Anna could be discharged home.

| CASE STUDY continued |

- Advocate for Anna to be admitted to a progressive and well-structured rehabilitation centre so that her progress can be as fast as possible.

- Explore the needs of the children: would they be better remaining with their grandparents who can provide for their physical and emotional needs; would there be a risk if they went to live with Anna that they would become the carers for their mother and then potentially have assessed needs of their own as young carers?

- Provide medication and/or cognitive behavioural therapy to deal with Anna's depression.

- Provide aids and adaptations to Anna's home.

- Arrange for an assessment under the NHS and Community Care Act (1990) and look into the possibility of direct payments to enhance Anna's sense of control over her services and utilise her intellectual capacity.

- Involve Anna fully in the decision-making process outlined above.

Analysis of the case study

In person-centred care, it is important to view people as individuals who are knowledgeable of their own conditions rather than adhering to the biomedical model (Ogden 2007), which perceives doctors and other health/social work professionals as the experts who 'know best' what an individual will need. In contrast, the biopsychosocial model of health (*ibid.* 2007) and the social model of disability place the responsibility for an individual's health, well-being and disability within a broader perspective, where professionals are challenged to include others, in this case Anna and her relatives, in the decision-making process related to an individual's present and future needs. In addition, the social model of disability challenges society to find different solutions to the problems that individuals like Anna might experience. Within this context, the following comments can be made about the case study:

- Treating Anna as a 'medical case', keeping her in hospital and performing a range of medical interventions may very slowly enable her to improve, but will certainly slow down her rate of recovery and make it more difficult for her to resume her roles as wife, mother and worker.

- Spending many months with Anna building up her skills and taking several hours a day to improve her ability to perform the tasks of daily living will promote her ability to do things on her own, but will leave her too exhausted to go out to work as she wants to do.

- Providing a service to assist Anna in undertaking some of her activities of daily living (Roper *et al.* 2000) will enable her to go home and fairly quickly resume her roles of mother and worker. In addition, it will be important for Anna to maintain her social and peer networks, which from a biopsychosocial perspective will be of great importance.

- In order to help further, interprofessional involvement will help to support Anna to achieve what she wants, with the consultant/general practitioner, occupational therapist, physiotherapist, care manager, social worker and nursing staff working together to ensure that the environment is as helpful as possible to achieve what Anna herself identifies as her goals and to enhance her own choices. While it is not always possible to meet the needs and wishes of all individuals, the key factor is to ensure that they are as fully involved as possible in the processes that contribute to decisions that affect their lives or their care (Koubel 2006).

- Some counselling or psychotherapy may help Anna to adjust to the changes in her life, particularly the loss of control over the various elements of her life rather, perhaps, than the loss of function. The issue of loss raises questions for professionals in their understanding of the impact of illness or disability.

- Anna may wish to utilise direct payments to provide a measure of control over whom she employs and what she actually wants them to do. However, if this proves too tiring and time consuming it may not be possible. It is possible that her parents could handle this at least initially, rather than actually taking on the care of the children.

- The children themselves may or may not need some help to adjust to the changes in their lives. Young carers are seen as people in their own right. It may be necessary for a social worker to assess that they are getting their needs met as children, but it is critical that this is seen as supportive to Anna and not as a signal that she is viewed as an incompetent mother purely because of her disability or impairment.

- There are issues that are not addressed overtly such as Anna's ethnicity, the involvement of her husband (the children's father) and the attitudes of her work colleagues to her disability and her ability to return to work. All of these need to be taken into account in a person-centred perspective.

This scenario raises many questions in terms of person-centred care and interprofessional working. There is always a risk in complex situations that the power of the combined interprofessional team, even where they are well meaning, can overwhelm the choices and wishes of the individual. All members of the team will need to be aware of their own potential to discriminate against the individual, even if this takes the form of thinking that they know what is best. These differences of opinion are not confined to the interprofessional team. There are a number of ways of attempting to understand the experience of an individual, some of which raise challenges for a person-centred, collaborative model of working. For example, as a consequence of their professional education and socialisation into their chosen profession, health and social care professionals will be likely to view the world of health and social care somewhat differently in terms of the types of interventions necessary.

Issues of loss (Currer 2007) and the individual's ability to 'adapt to that loss' are contentious in the disability movement. Within the discourse on the social model of disability, which clearly places the changes that are needed in the social arena (Oliver 1990) and questions whether the whole 'needs-led model of provision is inherently disempowering and segragationalist for disabled people' (Swain *et al.* 2005). Quinney (2006: 33) recognises that working in a collaborative way that closely involves the service user requires professionals to think in 'complex and dynamic models rather than simple linear models'.

Resources may be limited, but this does not mean that the cheapest option is best or necessarily the least effective. Trying to achieve what is actually wanted and keeping in mind the personal needs of the individual(s) involved is the best way to ensure that whatever resolution is achieved is the one most likely to succeed.

Too narrow a view of independence can be as limiting as too idealistic a view of society and the role of anti-discriminatory practice. Thompson's (2005) model for understanding the complex nature of discrimination is helpful, as it strives to encompass the realities of social and structural elements such as poverty, race and gender, while acknowledging the importance of the cultural differences (which may or may not be related to ethnicity) that will have an impact on the personal and psychological make-up of the individual. We have developed this further to encompass the make-up of the practitioners as well as the wider context for understanding the service user.

Person-centred care therefore fits quite comfortably with the values that underpin health and social care practitioners, but it also challenges them. This means that members of the interprofessional team have to be aware that person-centred care is not a simple concept, nor does it meet all the political or personal agendas of society or those who may seek health and social care interventions. The very concept of being someone who receives care is a difficult one in terms of people's feelings and their relationship with those who provide support or services. As Shakespeare (2000: 87) puts it: 'Help is collaboration, a shared participation in a common enterprise, but it involves a delicate balancing act, as with all moral action.'

Person-centred care must encompass the perspectives of individuals in all their varieties and complexities. Working interprofessionally with respect for each other's roles and expertise while maintaining the humanity and individuality of the individual at the heart of each intervention is a process that ethical frameworks, professional values and codes of conduct can help us struggle with (Banks 2001). Balancing this with the organisational pressures and political agendas is something that will continue to challenge us all.

References

Banks, Sarah (2001) *Ethics and Values in Social Work*, 2nd edn. Basingstoke: Palgrave Macmillan.
Bloy, M. (2002) The 1601 Elizabethan Poor Law, http://www.victorianweb.org/history/poorlaw/elizpl.html, accessed April 2008.

Brown, K. (ed.) (2004) *Vulnerable Adults and Community Care*, 2nd edn. Exeter: Learning Matters.

Centres for Disease Control and Prevention (2007) http://www.cdc.gov/, accessed: April 2008.

Currer, C. (2007) *Loss and Social Work*. Exeter: Learning Matters.

Data Protection Act (1998) http://www.opsi.gov.uk/Acts/Acts1998/ukpga_19980029_en_1, accessed April 2008.

Department of Health (2001) *Valuing Difference*. London: Department of Health.

Dominelli, L (2004) *Social Work: Theory and Practice for a Changing Profession*. Cambridge: Polity Press.

Elliott, P. (2003a) Recognising the psychosocial issues involved in hand hygiene. *Journal of the Royal Society for the Promotion of Health*, 123(2): 88–94.

Elliott, P.R. (2003b) Failing to adopt a patient centred approach: A multi-professional problem. *British Medical Journal*, http://www.bmj.com/cgi/eletters/326/7402/0#33297, accessed April 2008.

Elliott, P. (2006) Understanding clinical supervision: A health psychology orientated process of person-centred development. In M. Jasper (ed.) *Professional Development, Reflection and Decision Making*. Oxford: Blackwell.

Engle, G. (1980) The clinical application of the biopsychosocial model. *American Journal of Psychiatry*, 137: 535–44.

Festinger, L. (1962) Cognitive dissonance. *Scientific American*, 207: 93–102.

Health Protection Agency (2007) http://www.hpa.org.uk/, accessed April 2008.

Healthcare Commission (2007), http://2007ratings.healthcarecommission.org.uk/homepage.cfm, accessed April 2008.

Koubel, G. (2006) Decision making in professional practice. In M. Jasper (ed.), *Professional Development, Reflection and Decision Making*. Oxford: Blackwell.

Lawton, R. & Parker, D. (1999) Procedures and the professional: The case of the British NHS. *Social Science and Medicine*, 48: 535–61.

Lawton, R. & Parker, D. (2002), Barriers to incident reporting in a healthcare System. *Quality and Safety in Health Care*, 11:: 15–18.

Lorenz, K. (1994) *European Social Work*. London: Routledge.

Martin, S. (2004) *The Knights Templar: The History and Myths of the Legendary Military Order*. Harpenden: Pocket Essentials.

Moss, B. (2007) *Values*. Lyme Regis: Russell House.

National Health Service and Community Care Act (1990), http://www.opsi.gov.uk/ACTS/acts1990/ukpga_19900019_en_1, accessed April 2008.

Neuberger, J. & Tallis, R. (1999) Do we need a new word for patients? *British Medical Journal*, 318: 1756–8.

Ogden, J. (2007) *Health Psychology: A Textbook*, 4th. edn. Maidenhead: Open University Press/McGraw-Hill.

Oliver (1990) *The Politics of Disablement*. London: Macmillan.

Parker, D. & Lawton, R. (2003) Psychological contribution to the understanding of adverse events in health care. *Quality and Safety in Health Care*, 12: 453–7.

Quinney, A. (2006) *Collaborative Social Work Practice*. Exeter: Learning Matters.

Reason, J. (1998) *Human Error*. Cambridge: Cambridge University Press.

Reason, J., Parker, D. & Lawton, R. (1998) Organisational controls and safety: The varieties of role-related behaviour. *Journal of Occupational and Organisational Psychology*, 71: 289–304.

Rogers, C. (1961) *On Becoming a Person: A Therapist's View of Psychotherapy*. Boston, MA: Houghton Mifflin.

Roper, N., Logan, W. & Tierney, A. (2000) *The Roper-Logan-Tierney Model of Nursing: Based on Activities of Living*. London, Churchill Livingstone.

Roth, I. & Frisby, J. (1992) *Perception and Representation: A Cognitive Approach*. Milton Keynes: Open University Press.

Shakespeare, T. (2000) *Help*. Birmingham: Venture Press.

Singer, P. (ed.) (1994) *Ethics*. Oxford: Oxford University Press.

Swain, J., French, S. & Cameron, C. (2005) *Controversial Issues in a Disabling Society*, 2nd edition. Maidenhead: Open University Press.

Smith, M. (1998) *Social Science in Question*. London, Sage.

Southampton Centre for Independent Living (no date), *The Social Model of Disability*, http://www.southamptoncil.couk/social_model.htm, accessed April 2008.

Taylor, A. (2002), Global governance, international health law and WHO: Looking towards the future, *Bulletin of the World Health Organisation*, 80(12): 975–80.

Thompson, N. (2005) *Anti Discriminatory Practice*, 3rd edn. Basingstoke: Macmillan.

Thompson, N. (2007) *Power and Empowerment*. Lyme Regis: Russell House.

Wallston, K. & Wallston, B. (1982) Who is responsible for your health? The construct of health locus of control. *In* G. Sanders & J. Suls (eds) *Social Psychology of Health and Illness*. Hillsdale, NJ: Erlbaum.

Weinstein, N. (1984) Why it won't happen to me: Perceptions of risk factors and Susceptibility. *Health Psychology*, 3: 431–57.

Wilkinson, R. & Caulfield, H. (2001) *The Human Rights Act: A Practical Guide for Nurses*. Chichester: John Wiley & Sons Ltd.

PART

II

The Theory and Ethics of Person-Centred Care and Interprofessional Working

Person-Centred Care: With Dignity and Respect

Hilary Bungay and Rebecca Sandys

After the Second World War, Primo Levi, an Italian Jew who survived Auschwitz, wrote about his life in the concentration camp. Reflecting on man's inhumanity to other human beings, he asks us to consider how it feels to be deprived of everything and everyone that you care for and about:

> Imagine now a man who is deprived of everyone he loves, and at the same time of his house, his habits, his clothes, in short, of everything he possesses: he will be a hollow man, reduced to suffering and needs, forgetful of dignity and restraint, for he who loses all often loses himself.
>
> (Primo Levi 1958/1979: 33)

Although the passage refers to 'a man' it would equally apply to any one of us. What Levi seems to suggest is that without our loved ones, the ability to perform our usual daily tasks and our possessions, we lose our dignity and indeed our sense of self. To be able to practise person-centred care we need to have some understanding of what being a person means to us and others as individuals.

Therefore with this in mind, this chapter aims to challenge you to:

- Think about what being a person means to you.

- Consider when life begins and ends and how your conclusions may affect your practice.

- Define dignity, respect and autonomy and the factors that maintain or threaten an individual's dignity.

- Understand how dignity, respect and autonomy are intrinsically linked to being a person and person-centred care.

What is a person?

The established definition of a person is 'a human being regarded as an individual' (*Oxford English Dictionary* 2005), but in modern usage the term 'person' is subject to dispute and reinterpretation based on various perspectives. The Latin word *persona* was originally used to denote the mask worn by an actor. From this it was then applied to the role he assumed and, finally, to any character on the stage of life. As discussed in Chapter 2, personhood can be considered from scientific, sociological, philosophical (part of the 'humanistic circuit of knowledge') or theological perspectives.

Philosophers have debated the concept of personhood for centuries. Conceptually, a person may be defined by the characteristics of reasoning, consciousness and persistent personal identity. The English philosopher John Locke defined a person as:

a thinking intelligent being, that has reason and reflection, and can consider itself, the same thinking thing in different times and places; which it does only by that consciousness, which is inseparable from thinking, and as it seems to me essential to it.

(Locke 1689/1989 cited in Zagzebski 2001)

Another early definition is that given by Boethius in *De persona et Duabus Naturis*, where he defined a person as an individual substance of a rational nature. This definition also judges that the ability to reason is an essential part of being a person, which could be considered a good starting point. However, some philosophers have argued that a human being is purely a biological category, which does not take account of the psychological aspect and so disregards the mental or emotional components of personhood.

In the twentieth century philosophers and ethicists continued to argue and debate the characteristics of personhood. Singer (1979, 1995) suggested that persons have a particular significance or value because they have preferences and conscious desires that we can respect, and this determines both how we view others and the values we hold. Harris (1999), on the other hand, defines a person as a creature capable of valuing its own existence.

As we have seen from some of the definitions already considered, personhood is generally defined by a list of essential traits by which we recognise a human being as a person. Though these lists vary, they often include such characteristics as consciousness, the ability to reason, self-movement, self-awareness and a capacity to communicate. For sociologists though having a body with specific features, which has a certain place in society is necessary for us to recognise and identify a person (Turner 1996).

From the Christian theological perspective, personhood needs some relational interpretation of what it means to be a person. In this sense, personhood is often conceived of in terms of one's ability to have relationships with other human beings and the special relationship that human beings have with God. Campos (2002) describes the concept of personhood as neither logical nor empirical, but as an essentially religious or quasi-religious idea, based on one's fundamental (and therefore unverifiable) assumptions about the nature of the world.

Recognising these different perspectives we need to delve deeper, to explore basic concepts such as what being a person means to you. When does life begin or end and why do I think this? How might my belief affect my everyday practice? This chapter does not set out to instruct you as to what values or beliefs you should hold or even what is right or wrong, but rather to ask you to consider these questions and how they may affect your practice.

Personhood and person-centred care

Person-centred care (PCC), as we have seen in previous chapters, is a core notion in the context of health and social care provision. There is a universally recognised awareness of the positive aspects of introducing PCC into working lives (Rumbold 1993); Elliott and Koubel in Chapter 2 provide a detailed discussion of the concept of person-centred care in relation to interprofessional working. In the following sections a series of exercises are provided to assist you in formulating your own position as to what a person is, while considering the broader context and the viewpoints of others.

The implications of the conferral of person status for moral decision making in medicine, health care and research are complex. In medical and research ethics, three areas of ethical decision making in particular have been addressed through explorations into the conditions and criteria of personhood: the beginning and the end of human life and the morally relevant boundaries that separate human beings from nonhuman animals. According to Wiggins (1998), problems arise from the fact that the traditional concept of personhood is constituted by the three rather different ideas: the person as an object of science (biological, neurophysiological and so forth), as a subject of consciousness and experience, and as a locus of value and moral attributes.

Technologies such as test-tube pregnancies, implantable brain microchips, genetic engineering, cloning and robotics may well lead to changes in the human evolutionary process. If barriers between the species are blurred and blended through genetic engineering, how does this affect our notions of 'personhood'? Such factors will further influence our position on a range of health and social care issues, from the abortion debate to end-of-life decision making, to distribution of resources and also to animal rights. If traditional notions of personhood prevail, are we running the risk of denying essential basic liberties to sentient beings?

Attribute theories seek to differentiate a person from other animals. The most persuasive argument was propounded by Locke, as discussed above. One of the central themes that runs through the debate about the nature of a person is that a person possesses the ability to think and be rational. However, under this functional view a brain-damaged human being unable to demonstrate certain characteristics would fail to be acknowledged as a person. Conversely, using the argument that a person is able to think and be rational, could it be said that certain robots display these abilities? They too process information and their behaviour at times is convincingly intelligent. For example, Kismet (http://www.ai.mit.edu/projects/kismet/Kismet.QT3-T1-10f.mov) is a form of artificial intelligence. He does not have a proper body but he is able to interact with people, he displays and uses emotions, has feelings, is intelligent and is able to learn, and decides how to react to stimuli. In essence he is a baby and can do much that a five-month-old human can do. Barilan (2003) describes a human person as a sentient (thinking) being that is capable of experiencing pleasure, pain, frustration, satisfaction, memories and self-consciousness. Would you therefore describe Kismet as a person? Probably not, as there are other attributes that confer personhood. If we adopt a purely functional position that relies on an individual being rational and able to think, how would the concept of person-centred care apply to people in a persistent vegetative state or unconscious on an intensive care ward?

Another account defines the 'human person as an embodied mind' (McMahon 1999); that is, a human person is an individual with a body and a consciousness. But if having a body and a mind is necessary to be categorised as a person, how would we classify co-joined twins? They commonly share a body or body parts but have distinct personalities. In 2001 the Maltese co-joined twins Jodie and Mary were the subject of intense legal and ethical debate over whether they should be separated, as separation would mean the certain death of one of them, the debate centring on whether they were indeed two distinct people or persons (see Barilan 2003 for a detailed and thought-provoking examination of the surrounding issues). When we try to categorise an individual as a person, we could also consider patients with multiple personality disorders. Where there is more than one personality sharing one body, the mind cannot exist separately from the body; which personality owns the body that together makes them a person?

Who am I?

From the above statements we can see that although the answer to the question 'What is a person?' initially appears blindingly obvious, in reality it is a difficult and complex concept. Perhaps, then, we should consider it from a different perspective and ask ourselves: 'Who am I?' This is not just of academic interest: your conclusion will affect the way you think about key issues surrounding life, death and disability.

One way to do this is to consider the ways in which human beings are different from other animals. Genetics now tell us that we share 98 per cent of our genes with chimpanzees and 75 per cent with round worms. While at a genetic level we are remarkably similar to other creatures, there is evidence that chimpanzees and other primates do not have sufficient self-consciousness to be able to recognise themselves in mirrors (Gallup 1970 cited in Barresi 1999) and that they are only able to think in the here and now and do not have a sense of the past or future (Barresi 1999). It is our abilities to undertake such processes that make us distinct as persons from these other animals. However, if we extend this argument and use these features to distinguish between ourselves and chimpanzees, does this mean that we are not persons until we have a sense of 'self' and some concept of the future? Research has shown that young children typically do not have such awareness until the age of 4 (Barresi 1999). At that age children develop the ability to use a videotape of someone putting a sticker on their (the child's) head a few minutes earlier in the session to realise when the tape is replayed that the sticker might be still there and so remove it. Does this make children under the age of 4 or those without a sense of self non-persons?

So what makes you a person?

- Genetics?

- The ability to think?

- Self-awareness?

Some consider that human life begins at the moment of conception, but Harris (1999) argues against this view, on the basis that conception itself can result in a hydatiform mole, a cancerous multiplication of cells that will never become anything but a threat to the life of the mother. Furthermore, he argues that even if life does begin at conception it is not necessarily an individual life, but may form twins or triplets up to the 14th day afterwards. What is it about a human embryo or foetus that makes it distinct from other species, and makes it important to provide it with care, respect and resources? It may be suggested that it is the *potential* of the embryo to be born, to be human and to become an intelligent, self-conscious creature that makes it special. However, Harris dismisses this argument on two grounds: it is not inevitable that the embryo or foetus will become a functioning member of the adult human species; and at what point can a cell be said to have this potential? It is possible that any egg or sperm could achieve this at some point.

At the other of the spectrum at the end of life, medical technology's ability to maintain bodily functions in intensive care facilities also raises the question of the moment of death. Is a person who has no function in the cortical areas of his or her brain alive or dead? Some may claim that he or she is no longer a person, or that the person has ceased to exist, leaving only an 'empty shell'.

Forming an opinion about when a person's life starts influences our views on abortion and antenatal screening, including ultrasound where the foetus is clearly identified as a member of the human species. Likewise, our views on the end of life will affect how we view transplantation and switching off life-support machines.

Having thought about your own perspective on personhood, you can now decide what you think about such sensitive issues as:

- When do we become a person? *Conception, birth, aged 4?*

- When do we stop being a person? *Brain injury, death, coma, respiratory failure?*

At this point it may be helpful to use the who, what, when and where reflective template in Chapter 2 to consider 'What is a person?'. The different perspectives and opinions that may arise for you throughout this process may also help you to understand how complex some of the debates are around the allocation of treatments and resources. Moreover, it may help you to reflect on and understand why others may hold different views from your own.

Dignity, respect and autonomy

The principal foundations of personhood and person-centred care are individual dignity, respect and autonomy. The difficulty is to know how these principles can be integrated into our professions. Certainly in the UK the teaching of these terms has in the past been neglected, leaving a definite gap in the understanding and implementation of these core values by health care professionals (Department of Health 2003a). In the following sections, dignity, respect and autonomy will be considered in greater depth. However, once again it is not the purpose of the chapter to provide definitive definitions of these terms in relation to person-centred care, but rather to provide a spectrum of definitions and perspectives that allow you to decide for yourself what they represent to you and to come to an understanding that others' interpretations of these terms may differ and that meanings can change depending on life circumstances.

As a starting point, it is useful to look at the *Oxford English Dictionary* (2005) definitions. They are helpful because we can see how dignity and respect and autonomy are related:

■ *Dignity* originates from the Latin *dignitas*, from *dignus* meaning 'worthy'. It is the state or quality of being worthy of honour or respect, a composed or serious manner or style, a sense of pride in oneself, self-respect, a high or honourable rank or position.

■ *Respect* is defined as a feeling of deep admiration for someone or something elicited by their abilities, qualities or achievements; and due regard for the feelings, wishes, rights or traditions of others.

■ *Autonomy* originates from Greek *autonomos*, having its own laws, where *autos* means 'self' and *nomos* means 'law'. The autonomy of a country or region is the right or condition of self-government, freedom from external control or influence, and independence.

These definitions in reality demonstrate that dignity, respect and autonomy are actually quite vague abstract concepts. What do they actually mean? How could we explain these terms? Are dignity and respect the same; can you have one without the other? Before proceeding further try the following challenge.

=== **CHALLENGE** ===

Answer the following questions (adapted from Jacelon *et al.* 2004) and see whether you can define what 'dignity' means to you.

■ List all the uses of the word dignity that you can think of.

■ What are words that describe the opposite of dignity?

- How would you describe a person who is dignified?

- Is it desirable to have dignity or to be dignified? Why?

- How does a person become dignified?

- How would you describe a person who is not dignified?

- How can you give someone dignity?

- How can you measure dignity?

- How does our sense of dignity change with time?

- How can our sense of dignity change in different circumstances?

- Sum up in one sentence what having dignity means to you.

- Ask your family or friends what they think dignity is. Are their answers similar to your own views?

What is dignity?

Shotton and Seedhouse (1998: 246) suggest, 'It is tempting to think that dignity requires no definition. Anyone who has ever been in a degrading situation knows what dignity is: it is exactly what was lacking when it was most needed.' Within the health and social sciences literature there are many different definitions and ways in which people try and explain what dignity is (Griffin-Heslin 2005; Haddock 1996; Jacobson 2007; Matiti and Trorey 2004; Shotton and Seedhouse 1998). Although a number of definitions of dignity exist, in essence each fits within one of three distinct three levels:

- 'A certain quality which pertains to each and every person without each exception': the dignity attached to the whole human species.

- Self-respect: the dignity of human individuals.

- Social and political roles: the dignity of being part of a group within the human species (Feldman 2002; Szawarski 1986).

A quality that applies to everybody

The depiction of 'the dignity of the whole species' recognises that humans have special status: this gives us a basic dignity and we all possess it. It is essentially, fundamentally and irreducibly the dignity of being human. As early as the twelfth century the philosopher Alan of Lille defined a person as 'an individual distinct by reason of dignity' (Zagzebski 2001), and according to Szawarski (1986) 'being a person', 'being man' and 'having dignity' all mean the same.

This special status that we all hold is important when we are considering the allocation of health and social services, because from this definition we are all the same and should be treated equally, with no one person being judged to be more valuable than another. Zagzebski (2001) quotes the philosopher Kant, who contrasted dignity with price:

> Everything has either a price or dignity. If it has a price, something else can be put in its place as an equivalent; if it is excellent above all price and so admits of no equivalent, then it has a dignity.
>
> (Kant 1785/1958: 77)

Zagzebski interprets this as meaning that things with dignity cannot be compared in value to anything else, not even to other things with dignity. Dignity is therefore a part of all of us regardless of age, gender, status, race/ethnicity or religion.

Self-respect

Each person also has their own personal dignity and self-respect, which is dependent on many factors and varies over time. This 'dignity of identity' (Woolhead et al. 2004) is linked to respect and self-respect. Woolhead *et al.*'s study was part of a large project exploring the meanings of dignity with health care staff and older people, the Dignity in Older Europeans Project. In the study older people used examples to demonstrate how dignity of identity can be maintained or threatened. For example, it was suggested that drawing the curtains around a hospital patient's bed was a way of preserving the person's dignity; however, if conversations held behind the curtains could be heard by others through the curtains, then this could be as undignified as exposing the person physically. A person's dignity can be threatened by giving them a hospital gown that does not do up at the back, either because it is too small or is damaged, or wheeling them through a ward on a commode. Dressing older people in institutional clothing rather then their own is an assault on the 'self' because our clothes are often statements of our individuality. Likewise, allowing older cared-for adults to be seen in public with clothes incorrectly buttoned or dirty is degrading and threatens their dignity. Woolhead's study also found that autonomy and independence were important aspects of dignity: the capacity to have control. 'Toileting' everyone on a ward or in a care home at the same time was a threat to their autonomy and therefore their dignity. For all people personal dignity can change over time, and when people are dependent on others for care their own sense of personal dignity may be fragile.

Dignity associated with role or membership of a particular group

People also can possess (or lose) dignity through being a member of a group. This has to do with social and political roles where through holding a certain position the person involved acquires a special right to be respected. Traditionally, people in positions of power such as politicians, judges, the clergy and the medical profession have been given respect because of their status; some may argue that in modern society that this is an old-fashioned view. Indeed, are politicians still held in esteem, or have the numerous scandals involving them removed any special right to be treated with dignity and respect? Similarly with the clergy, as congregations reduce in size and the church has less of a role in people's lives, have they lost status in the community? In the modern day is 'celebrity' valued more? Is how we treat people dependent on their status? Do we treat someone with more dignity and respect because of their position; or with less dignity and respect because of how we perceive them, for example an older person or a drug addict?

- Who do you think has dignity?

- Why do you think this about them?

- How does this affect the way you think about them?

These three levels of dignity also have different dimensions. Matiti and Trorey (2004) describe dignity as being subjective, relative and evaluative. It is dependent on an individual's own assessment of dignity and so is subjective; it is therefore also relative because each person will perceive it differently; and because they arrive at their assessment through their own experiences it is evaluative. This means that the idea of dignity is often used to judge our own behaviour, how others behave and how others treat us.

What would threaten your dignity on an average day? Walking out of the lavatory with your skirt tucked into your pants or your flies undone? Slipping over in a busy shop, arguing with a friend or work colleague in a public place? Do these compromise your dignity or do they just make you feel foolish, something you would laugh about and then forget? Now consider the patient or service user who is already vulnerable through illness or personal circumstances: what threatens their dignity? Probably the same as the above, but what we as health and social care professionals do to them also has the potential to threaten or challenge their personal dignity.

When as part of the Dignity in Older Europeans Project (Arino Blasco *et al.* 2005), professionals were asked their views on dignity and what it means to treat someone with dignity, they provided the following responses:

- It implies treating them with courtesy and kindness, but it also means respecting their rights.

- Giving them freedom of choice.

- Listening and taking into consideration what they are saying.

- Being sensitive to people's needs and doing one's best for them.

- Involving them in decision making.

- Respecting their individuality.

- Allowing them to do what they can for themselves.

- Giving them privacy and their own personal space.

■ Treating an older person the same as everyone else, treating them as an adult and not as a child, treating them as part of the community.

Would you add any other point or action to this list?

CHALLENGE

Think about a care episode that you associate with the personal dignity of an individual at the receiving end of your care.

■ How did you help to maintain their dignity?

■ Was there anything that you did that could have been a threat to their dignity?

Respect

In policy documents dignity and respect are usually linked together, and in *Essence of Care* (Department of Health 2003b) dignity is defined as 'being worthy of respect'. Respect and self-respect are inherent components of dignity. Therefore we can see how interlinked dignity and respect are and that it is actually quite difficult to refer to one without the other.

In the *Agenda for Change* handbook (Department of Health 2007) there is a section on dignity in work that outlines the rights of people working in the NHS to be treated with dignity and respect, referring to the right not to be bullied or harassed. There is an expectation in interprofessional working that we will have respect for other disciplines' knowledge and the people with whom we work. There remains to some extent public respect for health professions and status associated with being a health professional: we are respected because of our roles and we have status bestowed on us by the position we have as gate-keepers, providers of care and the perceived value of the work we do. For social workers, however, there is not always the same level of public respect. Some may even describe themselves as being stigmatised, perhaps because the general public are unaware of the good work they do, particularly seeing reports in the media when things have gone wrong, sometimes with serious consequences. But as practitioners in health and social care we have a sense of self-worth and self-esteem from being a professional, having academic qualifications, employment, our role in the community, being a parent and our life experience. These contribute to our personal dignity. Similarly, the recipient of our care also holds personal dignity from their own employment status, family role and wider societal role, which we can support through respecting them.

Historically, when people required health care those who could afford it were seen by the family doctor, who knew the patient and their family circumstances. With evolving technology this therapeutic relationship between the patient/client and the doctor altered and instead of a 'sick person' the individual became seen and described as the 'gall bladder in bed eight' or the 'chest infection at no. 22'. The relationship between patients/clients and health and social care practitioners is again shifting with the introduction of person-centred care, the consumerist movement and such initiatives as the expert patient. People have become more knowledgeable about their health and also their rights; the use of the internet has widely disseminated information that at one time was only available to a select body of people, the 'professionals'. As the general public's knowledge has increased so respect for the professionals' body of knowledge has been eroded. Thus although generally speaking society respects us, there are increasing assaults on staff indicating a lack of respect, more litigation and less acceptance of 'doctor knows best'. All of this has an effect on the relationship between patients/service users and health and social care professionals.

We demonstrate respect for another person by how we act and what we say. Through person-centred care we show respect by recognising individual choice and personal boundaries, and through acknowledging the uniqueness of the person. According to Rushton (2007), respecting a person because they are a human being is different from respecting them for what they know, their position or their title. This links back to the different levels of dignity and suggests that we should not respect someone on the basis of their status or indeed consider them to be more or less dignified because of it. There are ways of preserving and maintaining a sense of respect while acknowledging the existence of human dignity. For example, staff on an intensive care unit will find out from the family about the lives of an unconscious person to help them to see the whole person and not just be treating the body, the illness or the disability (de Raeve 1996).

The use of people's preferred name rather than 'dear' or 'love' is very important in health and social care interactions, because failing to call someone by their proper name shows a lack of respect. It suggests either an unwillingness to be bothered to find out the person's name and how they wish to be addressed, or an inability to remember it.

People with learning difficulties or mental health problems may at times present a challenge for professionals in maintaining and demonstrating respect. However, Rushton (2007) believes that when we give another person respect, they experience a sense of worthiness. Nevertheless, respect is rather like dignity in that people are probably aware when they are not treated with respect, rather than registering that they have been given respect by someone involved in their care.

CASE STUDY: MRS BEGUM

Mrs Begum is a 78-year-old Bangladeshi woman whose ability to speak English is limited. She has been on an orthopaedic ward for some weeks recovering from complications following a hip operation. She has been unable to move around unaided, and has developed a bed sore on her buttock. One afternoon during visiting time, two members of the nursing team approach Mrs Begum, draw the curtains around her

---

CASE STUDY continued

bed and ask her to roll onto her side. She asks why and tries to explain that she is expecting visitors soon. One of the nurses says loudly, 'We want to have a look at your bottom.' It appears to Mrs Begum that everyone on the ward then goes silent and has heard what the nurse has said. She is very angry and distressed, and when her family visit later they are also very upset that she has been treated in this manner and would like to make a complaint.

CHALLENGE

- Imagine you are a member of Mrs Begum's family and write a letter to the ward manager summarising the complaint.

- The family members are unfamiliar with the complaints procedure. As a practitioner, how could you help them with this process? If you don't know, how would you find out?

- In responding to the complaint, are there any specific cultural or gender issues that the manager would need to take into account?

- As a manager, how would you a) respond to Mrs Begum and her family, b) approach the staff involved?

Autonomy

Autonomy is about the freedom to act and the freedom to decide for oneself, and again is linked to dignity. Indeed, for the philosopher Kant autonomy was the basis of the dignity of the human.

There are two types of autonomy: decisional and executional (Cardol *et al.* 2002). Decisional autonomy is perhaps what most people are referring to when they talk about 'respect for autonomy': it is the ability to make decisions. Within the health and social care professional and patient/client interaction there is inequality because the professional possesses a body of knowledge; which can make it difficult for someone who wishes to retain a level of control in their decision making. In order to make truly autonomous decisions people need to be given choices of possible treatment and/or care plans and these choices need to be genuine, which means that all the options are disclosed. Executional autonomy, on the other hand, is the ability to act on the basis of decisions. Evidently for some people with disabilities or illness executional autonomy is diminished and this can therefore affect their decisional autonomy, because the choices that are available to those without a disability or illness may be greater.

Just as dignity is a moveable concept so is autonomy. A person's autonomy may be restricted in the care environment. For example, an elderly person when living independently may get up every morning at 5 a.m. to make a cup of tea. If that person then enters a residential care home and is not permitted to do so, their freedom is restricted in much the same way as in institutions when all the residents are 'toileted' at the same time each day. However, respecting someone's autonomy also recognises their right to defer decision making to other people. Person-centred care means that we must respect a person's potential for autonomy during a care episode.

Van Thiel and van Delden (2001) describe four different perspectives on the understanding of 'respect for autonomy'. The liberal approach (Mill 1974) stresses the importance of independence and the freedom to make one's own choices, including the right to be left alone. There is the Kantian ideal of moral autonomy (Hill 1989), which requires that for individual decisions to be acted on or agreed to, the care giver must question the person's motivation for the choice. The narrative approach (Brody 1992) calls for the person's decision to be looked at in the context of their life, taking account of historical and cultural factors. Lastly, in the perspective of the ethic of care (Tronto 1993), independent decision making is not key; rather, decisions are made as a result of communication with all those involved in the caring relationship. Cardol *et al.* (2002) see the ethic of care as being an extension of the liberal view of autonomy that places a person's individual care needs and decision making within the context of their life narrative.

Whichever perspective you agree or disagree with, respect for autonomy necessitates empowerment through the provision of information, but also that decisions are made unhindered and independently without fear of reprisal.

CASE STUDY: MRS ELLIS

Mrs Ellis is on a rehabilitation ward after an operation following a fall at home. She would like to return home. At a multiprofessional team meeting to discuss her discharge, it is suggested to Mrs Ellis and her family that due to her condition she would be better going into residential care rather than returning home to live on her own. Mrs Ellis, supported by her family, wants to return home and to have visiting carers to assist her. After some discussion and negotiation, she complains that she is tired and wants to return to bed, but gives her family permission to continue the discussion with the team. The team and family agree that Mrs Ellis will return home with paid carers visiting three times a day to help her with the activities of daily living. The team stipulates that this arrangement will be continuously reviewed and a further team meeting will be called if she doesn't appear to be coping at home.

CHALLENGE

- In the case study, was respect for Mrs Ellis's autonomy demonstrated?

- Did the team adopt a liberal, moral, narrative or ethic of care approach to autonomy?

■ What were the potential threats to Mrs Ellis's autonomy?

■ Was this person-centred care? Give reasons for your answer.

Where do dignity, respect and autonomy fit with government policy on person-centred care?

It is only in recent years that 'dignity' and 'respect' have become established terms in government policy relating to health and social care services in the UK. Autonomy is less common, but issues around 'control', 'choice' and 'self-determination' are recurring themes in current policy and, as we can see from the above, are all components of autonomy. The concept of dignity became more prominent in law, policy and in the literature as a consequence of the atrocities conducted during the Second World War. In 1948, the General Assembly of the United Nations adopted and proclaimed the Universal Declaration of Human Rights. Article 1 of the Declaration states, 'All human beings are born free and equal in dignity and rights. They are endowed with reason and conscience and should act towards one another in a spirit of brotherhood' (United Nations 1948).

This was followed by the European Convention of Human Rights (1950), which was later enshrined in British law in the Human Rights Act 1998, aiming to protect all British citizens from actions that threaten their basic fundamental freedoms. Article 3 of the Act stipulates the right not to be subject to torture or to inhumane or degrading treatment or punishment. This is an absolute right and as such, under no circumstances are any exceptions permitted (Woogara 2004). For health and social care practice the significant phrase of Article 3 is 'inhumane or degrading treatment', because within the care environment there is the potential for patients and clients to be treated in a way that is both inhumane and degrading.

As health and social care practitioners in the UK we are governed by international conventions, government policy and our own professional codes of conduct, which aim to protect the people for whom we care. *The Patients' Charter* (Department of Health 1992) urged health workers to respect patients' 'privacy, dignity, and religious and cultural beliefs'. In *Modernising the Social Services* (Department of Health 1998) the importance of dignity for all service users was recognised. Later, *The NHS Plan* (Department of Health 2000) included a chapter called 'Dignity, security and independence in old age'. The following year the *National Service Framework for Older People* (Department of Health 2001) contained a chapter devoted to person-centred care that outlines the need for older people to be treated with dignity and respect. The Green Paper *Independence, Well-being and Choice* (Department of Health 2005) and the ensuing White Paper *Our Health, Our Care, Our Say* (Department of Health 2006a) set out proposals for the future of adult services and recognised the need for respect and dignity in maintaining independence, to allow people to achieve their potential and participate fully in community life. These proposals were all incorporated into *A New Outcomes*

Framework for Performance Assessment for Adult Social Care (Commission for Social Care Inspection 2006).

Service users and professionals worked together to describe good-quality care in order to try to change attitudes and promote new ways of working. As a result the *Essence of Care: Patient Focused Benchmarks for Health Care Practitioners* (Department of Health 2003b) was produced. This outlined a series of eight benchmarks for practice, one of which covered privacy and dignity and included seven factors recognising that patients benefit from care that is focused on respect for the individual (Table 3.1). Can you think of other examples of how dignity or privacy can be threatened?

Table 3.1   Potential challenges to privacy and dignity.

Factor	Benchmark of best practice	Examples of how privacy and dignity may be challenged
1 Attitudes and behaviour	Patients feel that they matter all the time	Staff discussing patients' treatment in their presence without acknowledging or involving them in the conversation
2 Personal world and personal identity	Patients experience care in an environment that actively encompasses individual values, beliefs and personal relationships	Removal of own clothes and personal belongings, lack of choice about where they are placed on a ward
3 Personal boundaries and space	Patients' personal space is actively promoted by all staff	Looking in patients' lockers without asking, entering the space around the bed when curtains are drawn without checking patient's state of dress
4 Communicating with staff and patients	Communication between staff and patients takes place in a manner that respects their individuality	Using terms of address use of 'love' or 'dear' or first name without permission
5 Privacy of patient, confidentiality of patient information	Patient information is shared to enable care, with their consent	Discussions taking place in shared bays when other patients or visitors can hear the conversation, notes being left open on nursing stations
6 Privacy, dignity and modesty	Patients' care actively promotes their privacy and dignity, and protects their modesty	Use of hospital gowns opening at the back and not be fastened, patient being wheeled through a ward on a commode
7 Availability of an area for complete privacy	Patients and carers can access an area that safely provides privacy	No access to a quiet room or garden

Source: Department of Health (2003) *The Essence of Care: Patient focussed benchmarks for health care practitioners*. London: Department of Health.

There are two noteworthy points about the benchmarks for privacy and dignity. First, although they were developed for the NHS and patients being cared for in a hospital setting, they are clearly as relevant to those working in the community either as health or social care professionals. It is just as easy to compromise a person's privacy and dignity in their own home as it is on a hospital ward. Secondly, it is difficult to say which of the benchmarks are specifically related to dignity and which are purely about privacy. Indeed, for some people privacy of the person and dignity are inter-related. For example, Woogara's (2004) definition of dignity incorporates many of the characteristics of privacy of the person: respect for the person, privacy of the body, privacy of space and territory, and having control over and choice of one's surroundings.

CASE STUDY: MISS PHILLIPS

Miss Phillips is middle-aged and has a learning disability. She lives at home with her elderly mother with support from social services. She recently had a fall and has an open wound on her thigh, which has been looked after and dressed by the district nursing team. Her social worker visits regularly and on this routine visit is accompanied by her supervisor. The social worker had previously worked as a nurse and had been unofficially monitoring Miss Phillips' wound, and had noted that the dressings on the wound sometimes appeared dirty and loose. Arriving at the house, the social worker lifted Miss Phillips' skirt and said to her supervisor, 'Look, this is what I was telling you about.'

When the visit had concluded the supervisor raised with the social worker the appropriateness of her behaviour. Why?

In 2006 the then Minister for Care Services Ivan Lewis launched the first ever Dignity in Care Campaign (Department of Health 2006b) aiming to stimulate a national debate around dignity and care. Its purpose was to create a care system where there is zero tolerance of abuse and disrespect of older people. It suggested that the absence of dignity in care is due to a combination of factors, including bureaucracy, staff shortages, poor management and lack of leadership, and deficiencies in training. Staff shortages and lack of time are often cited by staff when care or the lack of care becomes an issue, and yet relatively small changes to attitude, behaviour and practice can make a difference. It is interesting that such a campaign was instigated, particularly as the National Patient Survey for adult inpatients has consistently found that around 78 per cent of those asked whether they felt they were treated with respect and dignity while in hospital responded 'Yes always' (Health Care Commission 2004, 2005, 2006).

It is also of note that much of government policy surrounding the care of older people emphasises the need for them to be treated with dignity and respect. This does not mean that other groups in society do not deserve the same level of treatment, but perhaps rather reflects the perception that older people are more conscious of their dignity or may be seen as more vulnerable to losing their dignity? We then also need to consider what we mean by an 'older person'. According the Department for Work and Pensions, an older person is someone over 50 years of age. In its strategy for improving services for older and more vulnerable citizens, *Opportunity Age* (Department for Work and Pensions 2005), one of the core principles of service provision is that an older person is entitled to dignity, respect, freedom from abuse and good-quality care.

It is evident from the numbers of policies the government has produced that refer to dignity, and the introduction of a Dignity in Care Champions Network (Department of Health 2006), that dignity is considered a key issue for health and social care services. Yet, in addition to the driving force of government policy, health and social care professionals are already guided by their own professional codes of conduct. Examining a cross-section of these codes, it is apparent that there is a common theme extolling health and social care professionals to treat the people for whom they care with dignity and respect. *The International Code of Conduct for Nursing* (International Code for Nurses 1973: 63) states:

> Inherent in nursing is respect for life dignity and the right of man. It is unrestricted by considerations of nationality, race, creed, and colour, age, and sex, politics or social status.

The *Code of Ethics for Social Work* (British Association of Social Workers 2002) stresses that social work practice should promote respect for human dignity and that one of the basic values of social work is human dignity and worth:

> Every human being has intrinsic value. All persons have a right to wellbeing, to self-fulfilment and to as much control over their own lives as is consistent with the rights of others.

The *Code of Conduct and Ethics* (Society of Radiographers draft consultation 2007) maintains that members of the radiography workforce must:

> Treat all persons you come into contact with in professional and personal situations with respect and dignity irrespective of their gender, age, disability, ethnic origin, race, religion, beliefs, marital status, economic status, lifestyle, sexual orientation or political viewpoint.

The General Medical Council document *Good Medical Practice: Protecting Patients, Guiding Doctors* (General Medical Council 1998) states that it is necessary to respect patients' privacy and dignity to establish and maintain trust between doctor and patient.

These excerpts from codes of conduct and practice show that health and social care practitioners are working to common core values, which is essential in effective interprofessional working. We can see that internationally, nationally and at a professional level there is emphasis on dignity and respect. Yet despite the ideology of human rights having been with us since to middle of the twentieth century, there is still evidence of undignified treatment and abuses of elderly people and those with mental health problems or learning disabilities (Commission for Health Improvement 2003; Health Care Commission 2007). While such treatment reaches the headlines and is generally shocking to all who read about them, every day within health and social care individuals can be observed being treated with a lack of respect and in a manner that is undignified.

Removing or threatening someone's dignity can affect both the individual and society. At one level, it has been reported that the fear of loss of dignity is the reason most physicians give for those suffering a serious or life-threatening illness selecting or requesting euthanasia or some form of assisted suicide (Chochinov *et al.* 2002). At another level, according to Tadd *et al.* (2002) there is clear evidence that treating someone without dignity can impact on both treatment and social outcomes. From an economic perspective, treating people without dignity may result in complaints and even lawsuits, which have financial implications for the NHS and social services in dealing with such complaints. Tadd *et al.* (*ibid.*) also suggest that when judging treatment and levels of care, it is not just how clean the hospital is, its reputation and the expertise of its staff that influence how patients' visitors rate the standard of care, but how they see their relative and other patients being cared for in terms of simple everyday things such as how they are addressed, and whether they are in their own pyjamas or hospital gowns – in other words, whether the patients are perceived to be treated with dignity and respect.

Research has found that people who are hospitalised believe that dignity is something that can be taken away by others: that care and treatment can strip them of their dignity. On the other hand, outpatients and people in the community are more likely to feel that dignity is something you hold within you and so can't be taken away (Chochinov *et al.* 2002). Chochinov proposes that this could be due to outpatients having a greater degree of autonomy, whereas those who are hospitalised lose a sense of self. Their personal world and identity are threatened because they may not have their own clothes or belongings, and their own routine, which is individual to them, is also removed as they are required to conform to the ward routine. We can see therefore how the extract from Primo Levi at the beginning of the chapter can be used as a tool to help us realise how people may feel when hospitalised; although this is not to suggest that the experiences can be compared, as evidently the horror of internment is quite different to a stay in hospital. The important issue to take from this is the notion that removing people from their natural surroundings and taking away the factors that contribute to their sense of who they are can lead to a feeling of powerlessness, lack of control and loss of autonomy.

Conclusion

The concept of personhood and the question 'What is a person?' constitute for many people an intensely privately held belief. As health and social care professionals we may not hold the same beliefs as others but we can respect their views, while reflecting on the fact that philosophers, theologians and ethicists have been debating such concepts for centuries. The evidence indicates that policy makers, health and social care practitioners consider dignity and respect to be fundamental to the health and well-being of patients/clients/service users. If we are able to recognise the factors that can maintain or threaten a person's dignity and autonomy, it is likely that we will treat them appropriately and in a person-centred manner.

References

Arino Blasco, S., Tadd, W. & Boix Ferrer, J. A. (2005) Dignity in older people: The voice of professionals. *Quality in Ageing*, 6: 30–36.

Barresi, J. (1999) On becoming a person. *Philosophical Psychology*, 12: 79–98.

Barilan, Y. M. (2003) One or two: An examination of the recent case of the conjoined twins from Malta. *Journal of Medicine and Philosophy*, 28:1.

Boethius, C. *De persona et Duabus Naturis*, cited in *The Catholic Encyclopaedia: An International Work of Reference on the Church*, Charles George (1913), The Encyclopaedia Press.

British Association of Social Workers (2002) *The Code of Ethics for Social Work*. Birmingham: British Association of Social Workers.

Brody, H. (1992) *The Healer's Power*, New Haven, CT: Yale University Press.

Campos, P, (2002) Abortion and the rule of law. *Journal of Law, Medicine and Ethics*, 30: 4.

Cardol, M., De Jong, B. A. & Ward, C. D. (2002) On autonomy and participation in rehabilitation. *Disability and Rehabilitation*, 24(18): 970–74.

Chochinov, H. M., Hack, T., McClement, S., Kristjanson, K. & Harlo, M. (2002) Dignity in the terminology: A developing empirical model. *Social Science and Medicine*, 54: 433–43.

Commission for Health Improvement (2003) *Investigation into matters arising from care on Rowan ward, Manchester Mental Health and Social Care Trust*, Norwich: Commission for Health Improvement, www.chi.org.uk, accessed 14 September 2007.

Commission for Social Care Inspection (2006) *A New Outcomes Framework for Performance Assessment for Adult Social Care*. London: Commission for Social Care Inspection.

de Raeve, L. (1996) Dignity and integrity at the end of life. *International Journal of Palliative Nursing*, 2(2): 71–6.

Department of Health (1992) *The Patients Charter*. London: Department of Health.

Department of Health (1998) *Modernising the Social Services*. London: Department of Health.

Department of Health (2000) *The NHS Plan*. London: Department of Health.

Department of Health (2001) *The National Service Framework for Older People*. London: Department of Health.

Department of Health (2003a) *Choice, Responsiveness and Equity in the NHS*, London: Department of Health.

Department of Health (2003b) *The Essence of Care: Patient Focussed Benchmarks for Health Care Practitioners*. London: Department of Health.

Department of Health (2005) *Independence, Well-being and Choice*. London: Department of Health.

Department of Health (2006a) *Our Health, Our Care, Our Say*. London: Department of Health.

Department of Health (2006b) Dignity in care campaign, www.dh.gov.uk/PolicyandGuidance/HealthandSocialCareTopics, accessed 13 December 2006.

Department of Health (2007) *Agenda for Change Handbook, Version 2, NHS Employers*, London: Department of Health.

Department for Work and Pensions (2005) *Opportunity Age: Opportunity and Security Throughout Life*. London: Department for Work and Pensions.

Feldman, D. (2002) *Civil Liberties and Human Rights in England and Wales*, Oxford: Oxford University Press.

Gallup, G. G. (1970) Chimpanzees: Self-recognition. *Science*, 167: 86–7.

General Medical Council (1998) *Good Medical Practice: Protecting Patients, Guiding Doctors*. London: General Medical Council.

Griffin-Heslin, V. L. (2005) An analysis of the concept of dignity. *Accident and Emergency Nursing*, 13: 251–7.

Haddock, J. (1996) Towards further clarification of the concept 'dignity'. *Journal of Advanced Nursing*, 24: 924–31.

Harris, J. (1999) The concept of the person and the value of life. *Kennedy Institute of Ethics Journal*, 9(4): 293–308.

Health Care Commission (2004, 2005, 2006) *National Patient Survey*, London: Health Care Commission, www.healthcarecommission.org.uk.

Health Care Commission (2007) *Investigation into the Service for People with Learning Disabilities Provided by Sutton and Merton Primary Care Trust*. London: Commission for Healthcare Audit and Inspection.

Hill, T. E. (1989) The Kantian conception of autonomy. In J. Christman (ed.) *The Inner Citadel: Essays on Individual Autonomy*. New York: Oxford University Press.

International Code for Nurses (1973) *International Code for Nurses: Ethical Concepts Applied to Nursing*. Geneva: International Code for Nurses.

Jacelon, C. S., Connelly, T. W., Brown, R., Proulx, K. & Vo, T. (2004) A concept analysis of dignity for older adults. *Journal of Advanced Nursing*, 48(1): 76–83.

Jacobson, N. (2007) Dignity and health, *Social Science and Medicine*, 64: 292–302.

Kant, I. (1785) Groundwork of the metaphysics of morals. In Singer, P. (ed.) (1994) *Ethics*. Oxford: Oxford University press.

Kismet: http://www.ai.mit.edu/projects/humanoid-robotics-group/kismet/kismet.html, accessed 22 March 2007.

Levi, P. (1979) If This is Man: The Truce. London: Penguin. Originally published in Italy in 1958 as *Se questo è un uomo*.

Locke, J. (1989) *An Essay Concerning Human Understanding* Book 2, Chapter 27, Section 9. 1689. Ed. Peter. H. Niddick. Oxford: Clarendon Press.

Matiti, M. R. & Trorey, G. (2004) Perceptual adjustment levels: Patients' perception of their dignity in the hospital setting. *International Journal of Nursing Studies*, 41: 735–44.

McMahon, W. (1999) *Education and Development: Measuring the Social Benefits*. Oxford: Oxford University Press

Mill, J. S. (1974) *On Liberty*. London: Penguin.

Rumbold (1993) *Ethics in Nursing Practice*. London: Bailliere Tindall.

Rushton, C. H. (2007) Respect in critical care. *Advanced Critical Care*, 18(2): 149–56.

Shotton, L. & Seedhouse, D. (1998) Practical dignity in caring. *Nursing Ethics*, 5(3): 246–55.

Singer, P. (1995) *Rethinking Life and Death: The Collapse of Our Traditional Ethics*, Oxford: Oxford University Press.

Singer, P. (1979) *Practical Ethics*. Cambridge: Cambridge University Press.

Society of Radiographers (2007) *Code of Conduct and Ethics*, draft for website consultation, www.sor.org.uk, accessed 24 July 2007.

Szawarski, Z. (1986) Dignity and responsibility. *Dialetics and Humanism*, 2–3: 193–205.

Tadd, W., Bayer, T. & Dieppe, P. (2002) Dignity in health care: Reality or rhetoric. *Reviews in Clinical Gerontology*, 12: 1–4.

Tronto, J. C. (1993) *Moral Boundaries: A Political Argument for an Ethic of Care*. New York: Routledge.

Turner, B. S. (1997) *The Body and Society*. London: Sage.

United Nations (1948) *The Universal Declaration of Human Rights*, adopted and proclaimed by General Assembly resolution 217 A (III) 10 December 1948. New York: United Nations.

van Thiel, G. J. M. W. & van Delden, J. J. M (2001) The principle of respect for autonomy in the care of nursing home residents. *Nursing Ethics*, 8: 419–31.

Wiggins, D. (1998) *Needs, Values, Truth: Essays in the Philosophy of Value*. Oxford: Oxford University Press.

Woogara, J. (2004) Patients' right to privacy and dignity in the NHS. *Nursing Standard*, 19(18): 33–7.

Woolhead, G., Calnan, M., Dieppe, P. & Tadd, W. (2004) Dignity in older age: What do older people in the United Kingdom think? *Age and Ageing*, 33: 165–70.

Zagzebski, L. (2001) The uniqueness of persons. *Journal of Religious Ethics*, 29(3): 401–23.

Self-Awareness: The Key to Person-Centred Care?

Claire Barber, Niall McLaughlin and Janet Wood

This chapter aims to demonstrate how effective person-centred care and inter-professional working are a product of:

- Self-awareness.

- Verbal and non-verbal communication skills.

This chapter also aims to develop an understanding of how these are informed by:

- Culturally entrenched professional norms.

- The way our values consciously and unconsciously affect our perceptions of others.

Care is delivered through human interactions between the practitioner and the service user. This chapter promotes the concept that care cannot be effective unless learners can develop a concept of themselves as professionals and service users as persons by:

- Enabling health and social care learners to consider how self-awareness as a practitioner is a crucial aspect of person-centred care.

- Promoting the concept that the practitioner's beliefs and perceptions of others affect the delivery of person-centred care.

The Johari Window offers the reader a model through which to increase self-awareness. The obstacles to self-awareness are considered alongside the opportunities for personal development that are offered by practice placements. Practice examples are analysed for their therapeutic impact and to promote reflection on the barriers to and opportunities for person-centred care. In addition, a review of key frameworks on the origins of person-centred practice are presented, including:

- The therapeutic self and Rogers' core conditions of genuineness, acceptance and empathy.
- Beliefs, values and the impact of labelling.
- Barriers to person-centred care.

Health and social care professionals and learners are asked to consider through working examples how in their role as practitioners they can promote person-centred care in their communication with service users and other professionals. Reflecting on critical questions creates an increasingly rich dialogue for self-development and this chapter aims to enable health and social care learners to begin to take responsibility in asking critical questions of themselves. For some, developing this understanding may involve the deconstructing and rebuilding of long-held values and reconciliation with 'hidden' aspects of personality. The chapter concludes, therefore, with an exploration of the rationale behind this approach and the articulation of the underpinning philosophy of individualised, humanistic values in health and social care.

Introduction

Practitioners in health and social care endeavour to attain an increasingly inter-professional and person-centred delivery of services and they may advance towards these goals along separate paths. Usefully, this can accommodate different rates of progress. Nevertheless, there are on many journeys points at which all paths converge to traverse a challenging terrain.

Preparation for interprofessional practice offers an opportunity for each practitioner to define her or his self. Likewise, it is only through a person-centred approach that those whose recovery we seek to promote can arrive at a definition of well-being that is personally meaningful. While only the service user can ultimately determine their own level of well-being, each practitioner will have a concept of what it means to be well. This concept will be informed by their professional perspective and by their personal values. A mental health nurse may, for example, be inclined to arrive at a definition based on subjective reporting of values such as happiness or fulfilment. An operating department practitioner, however, may also be able to draw on more quantitative data, such as heart and respiratory rates. Therefore, not only do practitioners need to adopt a person-centred approach in order to arrive at a meaningful description of well-being, it is also incumbent on them to look beyond traditional professional boundaries if a holistic definition is to be attained. That these are fundamental questions of personal identity may be disputed by those who would argue that it is sufficient for the service user to be 'treated as a person' and for the practitioner to 'act professionally'. This approach has neither proven historically to be an effective safeguard against abuse, nor will it offer scope for further improvement of services.

The philosophy of person-centred care has developed in response to the need for a more user-sensitive health and social care service and is based on a rich understanding of the person's circumstances and needs (see Elliot and Koubel, Chapter 2). Price (2006) adds that this is a concept that has been 'big in intent but limited in practical application' and that to become a practical reality, person-centred care must be interpreted in the context of service user and organisational circumstances.

Organisations and professional groupings need to adopt more holistic approaches in order to support the service user's progress towards well-being and to do this need to develop interprofessional models of care delivery. However, traditional affiliations may prove hard to overcome unless professionals are prepared for such developments. Many practitioners will acknowledge that their choice of career was influenced by an idea of the type of person they considered themselves to be. Many will also acknowledge changes in their personality connected with their professional role. Practitioners need to look within themselves to recognise the narrowing influence that the traditional distinctions between these groupings might have on their value base. However, each person's set of values pre-dates and continuously informs their professional identity.

Self-awareness

If human interactions are central to effective person-centred care and a broad personal and professional perspective is essential to holism, then it follows that development of practitioner self-awareness is crucial. An awareness of who we are as a person in professional practice can help not only to illuminate how we view and respond to others, but also how others view and respond to us as practitioners.

The Johari Window can show us that those aspects of ourselves for which the way we think of ourselves corresponds closely with the way others think of us may only be a small part of our 'personality' as a whole:

- *Open area* – What a person knows about him- or herself and is prepared to share with others: the 'public self'. Can also include clothes worn, expressions, what others see. Do you wear an ID badge or uniform – how much does it reveal about you? Do you use a store card or loyalty card?

- *Hidden self* – What a person knows about him- or herself but is inclined not to disclose: the 'private self'. This includes fears, doubts, anxieties, fantasies, feelings of conflict and confusion, dreams and ambitions.

- *Blind self* – What others may know about a person but that person may not know personally. Are you secretly envious of or irritated by another person

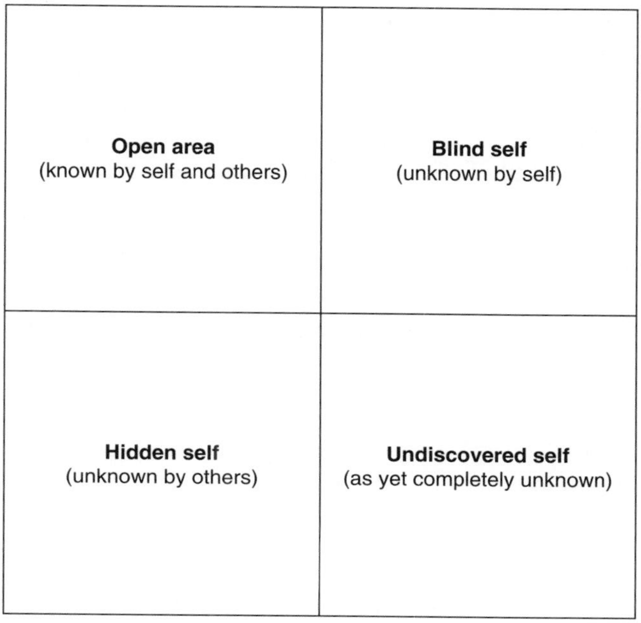

Open area (known by self and others)	**Blind self** (unknown by self)
Hidden self (unknown by others)	**Undiscovered self** (as yet completely unknown)

Figure 4.1 Johari Window.

Source: Based on Luft, J. & Ingham, H. (1955) The Johari window: A graphic model of interpersonal awareness.
Proceedings of the Western Training Laboratory in Group Development. Los Angeles, CA: UCLA.

but never told them? There's a good chance somebody else feels the same way about you.

■ *Undiscovered self* – at least consciously to the person or other people: the 'unknown self'. This is difficult to access, but you may get a hint of this through 'slips of the tongue' or non-verbal leakage. One way of looking at this might be to think about situations not yet experienced and anticipate how you might respond to them, e.g. cardiac arrest, involvement in a child protection situation, breaking bad news.

The Johari window (cited in Chapman 2006) was developed by psychologists Joseph Luft and Harry Ingham in the 1950s as a tool to aid self-awareness. The window can help us learn intrapersonal skills that can have a profound effect on our ability to communicate with others effectively (interpersonal skills) in order to become more effective practitioners. The Johari window involves consideration of that which is 'known to self' and, conversely, 'unknown to self'; also what is 'known to others' and 'unknown to others'.

The window is divided into four equal parts. However, through the use of reflective thought it is hoped that the areas that are 'unknown' prior to reflection decrease in size, allowing more room for openness. The process of exploring each quadrant can develop our understanding of ourselves and of how we can overtly use aspects of our personality to communicate in a genuinely robust and meaningful way. In order to use this tool it is necessary to acknowledge that two perspectives exist: your perspective and the perspective of others. There will be times when knowledge of self does not correspond with that of others. There may also be instances when we deliberately decide to withhold or not share certain aspects of our private self. Equally, there may be occasions when it is the practitioner who is in the dark in terms of not knowing an aspect of their personality that others may be able to see or feel. In clinical situations there may also be times when a person, in an acute phase of their illness, may not be willing to participate in their treatment. It is necessary to develop an empathetic appreciation of the person's illness, their individual experience of the illness, the service and their treatment.

Practising in a person-centred way involves consideration of the contextual issues and the individual's symptomatology. Reflecting on such matters can shed new light on intrapersonal and interpersonal knowledge that is crucial to becoming an autonomous, insightful practitioner. Our experiences of caring for people can therefore be directly changed by our involvement in self-reflection, producing appreciative communication and clarity of reason in person-centred interventions. Person-centred care should not be just a philosophy or policy-driven rhetoric; it needs to be action oriented and begin with each student or practitioner taking responsibility for their own practice.

=================================== **CHALLENGE** ===================================

Create your own Johari Window illustrating it with examples from your practice. If you're feeling brave, you might want to seek feedback from a colleague, friend or family member to help you fill in the 'blind self'.

■ What are the processes by which aspects of ourselves may move from one area of the window to another?

■ Are some kinds of self-awareness easier to obtain than others?

■ Try doing the window with a work colleague and then a family member or friend. Does the window change? Why do you think this is?

Communications theory

The balance between the aspects of ourselves described by the Johari Window may be continually changing, but this is not to dismiss the notion that we may have core personal and professional values or that we may be 'comfortable' with who we are. Assuming, then, that we have a 'professional identity' and that this is broadly functional, there is still no guarantee of how we might be perceived by others. A degree of insight into and, ultimately, control of this process can be established nonetheless by attending to the processes by which such perceptions are formed.

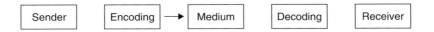

Interpersonal communication between two people has as its building block the transfer of information [a message] from one person to the other.

The person sending the information will have an idea of what they want to convey. They will convert this idea into words and actions – a process referred to as 'encoding'. These words and actions will be carried by sound and sight [known as the media] to another person who will then transform [decoding] them into an idea in their own mind. (Dimbleby & Burton 1998)

In the real world things are often not so simple – the phrase 'a cry for help' is often applied to an episode of self-harm or attempted suicide. The premise of such a description is that the sender has specifically *not* cried for help, but has encoded their message as a destructive act against the medium of their own body.

At each stage between the forming and receiving of any message there is the possibility of interference, which may hinder the communication process. Obvious examples of interference might include background noise in a care environment, a phone call that 'breaks up', a poor-quality printout or illegible handwriting.

The problems that affect interpersonal communication are well exemplified by the game Chinese Whispers, but even this pre-supposes a desire by the participants to communicate effectively. However, in complex health and social care situations this cannot always be assumed on the part of the professional or the recipient of care. There are many important social care and health issues that we 'don't want to talk about': debt, sexual activity, how we discipline our children, continence to name but a few. There may also many reasons why we 'just don't want to hear it': if we haven't the time, have run out of patience or don't want to learn that our efforts were in vain.

Interference that affects the competence of the medium to carry the message accurately can be more easily identified and remedied than that which affects the ability of the sender to encode or the receiver to decode. This latter category may then be further subdivided into those sensory factors that affect the encoding and decoding, and finally into those psychological factors that affect the way in which we interpret and represent our experiences.

CHALLENGE

Apply the model of communication to a care situation from your own professional speciality.

- What factors might impair the message?

- What can the professionals do to promote effective communication?

- Consider communications with other professionals. What are the barriers to effective communication?

Perception

Consider both of the pictures in Figure 4.2. Each can be seen in three ways. The picture on the left, for instance, can be seen as:

- A saxophonist.
- A woman's face.
- Or both.

In any large group of people there will be some who see only the saxophonist and some who see only the woman. If you can see only one face in the right-hand picture, try asking someone to show you the other. In this moment you may feel your brain resisting a truth that is in front of your eyes.

What these optical illusions tell us therefore is:

- What we see when we look at something may not be the same as what another person sees.
- Sometimes as soon as we think we know what we are looking at our brain tells our eyes to stop looking (Hochberg 1972 in Gombrich 1972).

The consequences of this phenomenon extend directly into health and social care situations, for instance:

- Looking at an X-ray or scan image and seeing a large fracture or shadow but not seeing an additional, smaller one.
- Reading a client's case notes, picking out the words that match our preconceptions and rejecting other data.

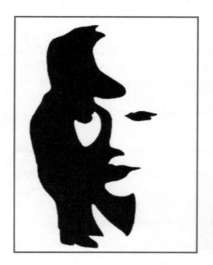 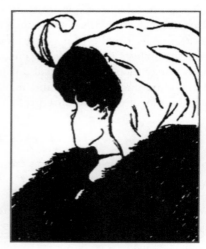

Figure 4.2 Optical Illusions.

If this can happen when we look at an image or read text, it might also occur with any of the senses we use when we encounter a person so, potentially:

■ Any ideas we have about other people might not be the whole picture.

■ We might be wrong about what other people think about us.

■ Other people might be making inaccurate assumptions about us.

It has already been considered, via the Johari Window, that there are things we don't know about ourselves and others and that others have different impressions of us from those we imagine. If it can be demonstrated additionally that we have the capacity to jump to conclusions about things like pictures (which we presumably approach without any preconceived notions), it seems likely that were we to encounter real people with ready-made assumptions about what they might be like, or were we to carry into these encounters ideas about the sorts of people that there are in the world, then we are even more likely to jump quickly to inaccurate conclusions about them.

To consolidate the ideas expressed so far in this chapter, a scenario is offered in which a client's contact with services is represented in five varying accounts, each offering different perspectives.

CASE STUDY

1. Mr D. was vague about the details of the overdose. Apparently he took 100 tablets the day before he presented himself to the hospital. He said he had 'no idea' why and 'can't remember'. He was alone at home at the time and drank three cans of strong lager after the O/D. Later in the day he was arrested for drink-driving. He only sought help 24 hours later for back pain. Mr D. told me he often O/Ds and cuts himself in order to deal with his distress – but rarely with suicidal intent.

2. Over the last six years Mr D. has had many episodes of deliberate self-harm – cutting and overdosing. He has attended A&E numerous times and has lived out of the area for the last two years. He said he's been admitted twice for detox, however his wife told me he'd been detained under the Mental Health Act. He has a long history of alcohol abuse and has cirrhosis of the liver.

3. David was born in Newcastle. Removed from alcoholic parents at a few weeks old. Grew up in care and from 5 years old was abused physically, sexually and emotionally. He says his mother died through self-neglect and alcoholism and that he has two sisters who he has never met and three brothers of whose where abouts he is no longer aware. As a teenager he left care and went straight into Borstal. He served several years in jail for drug-related offences. 15 years ago he found a friend dead from a drug overdose, which shocked him into stopping his own drug

use. He found regular employment and married and describes himself as 'happy' for these 10 years. He most recently worked three years ago. He has a 10-year-old son to his wife and lives on a caravan park close to her and her two other sons.

4. A 43-year-old gentleman. Six years ago, his son was abused along with many others at a local authority nursery. While he had been able to cope with his own memories, the subsequent inquiry brought these to the fore. Over the last six years he has cut himself and overdosed on many occasions. He does this to distract himself and relieve his emotional distress. He describes himself as feeling on a 'high' after he has self-harmed. He also drinks an average of five cans of 5% lager a day.

5. A thin, unkempt man. Poor self-care. Mood variable. Sleep varies according to alcohol intake. Appetite diminished. Eats once daily with his family and has lost two stone over the past few months. No particular anxieties or concerns. No evidence of disordered thinking. Some visual disturbance but no clear hallucinations. Dislikes and avoids busy places and crowds. Keeps himself socially isolated. With regard to future was very negative – says he will take 'one day at a time'. He thought it inevitable that he would harm himself again.

CHALLENGE

■ Who might have written these different accounts?

■ What are the characteristics of the accounts that offer the most complete picture?

■ Do some of the terms used in the account prompt negative thoughts about David's entitlement to services?

■ Would the way you worked with David be affected by what you read about him beforehand?

■ Could you make an accurate clinical decision based on any single account?

■ What are the long-term prospects for David if the professionals involved don't share their information with each other?

Only if the professionals in this case communicated with each other did they have a chance of developing an effective plan for the man's support and recovery.

The consequences of the possibility that our perceptions of a person can be so seriously distorted by both our personal value systems and by role-restricted professional practices is now considered from the perspective of first interprofessional working and then the practitioner-service user relationship. Finally, options are offered for exploring these issues further through tools and case studies aimed at enhancing reflective practice.

Interprofessional practice

Findings of high-profile inquiries in a diversity of settings, such as the Laming Report (2003) into the death of the child Victoria Climbie and the Ritchie inquiry (Ritchie et al. 1994) into the care and treatment of mental health service user Christopher Clunis, have highlighted the lack of inter-professional communication and information sharing as a contributory factor to these tragedies. This has led to contemporary government policy and guidelines, such as the National Service frameworks for Mental Health (Department of Health 1999), Older People (Department of Health 2001) and Children (Department of Health 2004), requiring that health and social care agencies work together collaboratively in order to enhance service provision. More recent policies, including the Report on Adult Care Services (Beresford et al. 2005), have added impetus to this requirement. However, there are challenges that need to be considered if professionals are to work together effectively. Hornby and Atkins (2000) identify a number of barriers to interprofessional collaboration, including rivalry, mismatch in terminology and lack of trust. If such barriers are not acknowledged and dealt with, then interprofessional working is unlikely to achieve the required person-centred outcomes. As Leathard (2003) observes, when interprofessional approaches work well they have inherent qualities that can benefit decision making and working practices.

Herbert (2005: 2), defines collaborative patient-centred practice as 'a practice orientation, a way of healthcare professionals working together with their clients to enhance service user and family centred goals and values' In this model of interprofessional working, the active participation of each discipline in clinical decision making is promoted both within and across disciplines. As multidisciplinary, community-based services are being required to engage with ever more complex health and social care problems, a benefit of interprofessional practice (Copperman & Newton 2007) is that different perspectives, knowledge bases, values and skills lead to an enhanced capacity to solve these problems. There is also evidence (Hall *et al.* 2007) that such models of collaborative working can not only enhance person-centred care but may lead to more satisfying work roles for practitioners.

It can be argued, then, that to deal with the barriers to interprofessional working and capitalise on opportunities for person-centred care, an awareness of who we are in professional practice is imperative. As Meads and Ashcroft (2005: 27) point out, 'collaboration is, in part a personal decision and is as much about who the individual is as about what they do'.

Have the health and social care roles that have traditionally developed around discrete units of care equipped us for this changing environment? On the positive side, it is possible that strong professional identities offer a clarity that facilitates informed choice by a service user: a service user in the community may find it helpful to understand that they need to discuss their medication with a nurse, their benefits with a social worker and their accommodation with a housing manager, for example. These distinctions are only useful to the extent that the service user has access to all these professionals. In situations where access is, at best, often limited to only one community professional, then this professional becomes a very powerful 'gatekeeper'. This gatekeeping role is readily represented in terms of access to services, but it applies equally to the way in which the needs of the service user are represented to others. The situation resulting from this would therefore be that professionals removed from traditional roles and given – as human beings – to forming rapid opinions about new situations are being required to communicate, with care outcomes being dependent on their personal and professional judgements.

The example of David illustrates the hazards inherent in using information from a limited range of sources and also shows that there is often a fine line between the deployment of professional terminology and the stigmatising use of pejorative labels.

Labels

Person-centred care has been defined as 'valuing people as individuals' (Winefield *et al.* 1996). However, one study (Coyle & Williams 2001) found that patients' sense of individual identity had been threatened by some experiences of healthcare services that they perceived as dehumanising, objectifying, disempowering and devaluing. Although many patients also expressed positive experiences of care in this study, it does bring into question the extent to which people felt that some service practices valued them as individuals.

The concept of labelling has been explored by many authors since, but arguably the seminal work was conducted by Erving Goffman (1963), who wrote, 'Labelling is a means to describe and categorise objects and helps us to make sense and order of the world around us.' Goffman extends the meaning to describe the process by which people are designated by some behaviour that society deems deviant. This can often carry pejorative connotations, such as those for 'homeless', even when we know that most homeless people do not occupy that position in society through choice.

Labelling is a two-way process: the person labelling has one set of responses; the person labelled has another set, which can be embraced or rejected by the subject of the label. Labels can be both a means of subjugation and a source of empowerment at the same time. There are a number of racial epithets that are used in both ways.

Professional job titles offer labels that bespeak more than a mere description of the role. How informative is the answer 'social worker' or 'nurse' to the question 'What do you do for a living?'. How often does it elicit a response – even from other health and social care professionals – such as 'I couldn't do your job!'? The label doesn't in any way describe our day-to-day professional activities and it is likely that even others within health and social care have only a sketchy idea of our practice. That the label and the response are understood as having conveyed meaning indicates that if boundaries between groupings are to be diminished, such perceptions need to be examined and challenged. Implicit also in the response 'I couldn't do your job!' is an appraisal of the personality of the health and social care professonal: that they have courage, a strong stomach, resilience in the face of human suffering, or (perhaps negatively) that the respondent is a more sensitive person.

Stereotypes

Clusters of characteristics are attached to specific labels and these characteristics are often attributed to the personalities of those people to whom the label applies. Think of 'There was an Englishman, an Irishman and a Scotsman...' A joke in this format shared between English people almost inevitably makes negative assumptions about the Scots and the Irish, which must be unspoken for the joke to function.

Despite the apparently overwhelming evidence that stereotyping is negative in its effects, without this way of thinking about people and things we simply couldn't function, because not only would every new situation overwhelm us, we would also have no ideas about ourselves and how we are supposed to act. As well as defining others we define ourselves in these ways:

- I'm a nurse.

- A Sikh.

- A vegetarian.

- A mother.

- Environmentally conscious.

- A party animal.

This taxonomy of characteristics helps us to orientate ourselves quickly and respond consistently, so we cannot abandon labels and stereotypes.

> Our past experiences, current circumstances and future hopes and expectations all contribute to our feelings, attitudes and beliefs. These in turn affect what we do, what we notice about and how we interpret other people's behaviour.
>
> (Kagan *et al.* 1995: 6)

Hence we return to the concept of awareness. Self-awareness will help us to work sensitively and constructively with the deployment of labels and stereotypes by us and about us. Awareness of the concept itself will help us to break down barriers to interprofessional and interpersonal communication.

Stigma

We may be happy with certain stereotypes until a change occurs or we encounter adverse conditions. However, health and social care professional roles often lead to encounters with service users whose wider circumstances are perpetuating their problems and who require support in a change process. We are required therefore to look beyond the sort of labels that may have been attached to a service user with whom we are working. The extent to which people feel valued as individuals by others is critical to having a positive sense of self. According to Byrne (2001), to be marked or labelled as, for instance, 'mentally ill' carries both internal (secrecy, lower self-esteem and shame) and external (social exclusion, prejudice and discrimination) consequences for the person. These consequences are collectively understood as 'stigma'. Individuals with a label of mental illness have been subject to negative stereotyping in public domains such as the media that are associated with characteristics of unpredictability, incompetence and dangerousness (Hayward & Bright 1997; Repper & Perkins 2005; Summerfield 2001). There is evidence that negative stereotypes such as these perpetuate myths that influence not only public perceptions, but also those of practitioners. One study based on the experiences of UK mental health service users found that 70 per cent had experienced discrimination in some form: 47 per cent in the workplace, 44 per cent from general practitioners and 32 per cent from other health care professionals (Wright & De Porte 2000).

Negative stereotypes and attitudes such as these result in discrimination that can affect all aspects of day-to-day living, including employment, relationships, income, access to services, family life and parenting (Repper & Perkins 2005; Social Exclusion Unit 2004). These experiences can have a huge impact on how people labelled as mentally ill view come to view themselves and their capabilities:

> When I was diagnosed I felt 'this is the end of my life.' It was a thing to isolate me from other human beings. I felt I was not viable unless they found a cure… I felt flawed, defective.
>
> (cited in Sayce 2000)

This experience of feeling 'different', 'flawed' and 'defective' can both arise from and be reinforced by the medical model with its focus on diagnosis, deficits and dysfunctions based on assumptions of a biological origin to mental illness (Chadwick 1997). This suggests that a more holistic, person-centred care approach can be viewed in contrast to the medical model and at times a tension between these approaches may occur (Jones 1999). In one study of young men recovering from psychosis (Lloyd et al. 2005), the effects of labelling and stigma on interpersonal relationships and the changes in self-perception that these effects bring were clearly evidenced.

The process of labelling people in health and social care services can give rise to individual and organisational responses based on negative stereotypes and perceptions that may be contrary to the principles of person-centred care. This is especially true for service users and their families, who may be labelled as 'difficult', 'manipulative' or 'non-compliant'. It is often those who are engaged in potentially risky lifestyles and behaviours (homelessness, substance misuse, self-harm) that are recipients of these sorts of labels and responses.

In one study exploring 'non-compliance' in health care (Russell et al. 2003), it was proposed that practitioners' dominant view of this issue fails to take account of the social context of people's lives. In an alternative social view, non-compliance is not simply a matter of service users choosing not to follow advice, but it is recognized that choice may be constrained by individual life-styles and social circumstances. In a person-centred care approach these wider social circumstances need to be considered and the practitioners' discomfort that may be related to non-compliance recognised and addressed, rather than resorting to defensive and distancing responses such as negative labelling and stereotyping of individual service users and families. (The term 'compliance' has fallen out of favour as it considered pejorative and the word 'concordance' is now used in preference. However, where 'non-compliance' has been used in the research referred to throughout this chapter we have retained it in accordance with the original authors' usage.)

So, practitioners use labels and stereotypes to dissociate themselves from the adverse outcomes of interventions and this may be one way in which we protect ourselves from the stressful experience of working with vulnerable people in difficult circumstances (Obholzer & Roberts 1994). Paradoxically, the evidence above suggests that such strategies are increasing the likelihood of adverse outcomes. It follows from this that an engagement with service users in which we consciously deploy our *selves* as the agents of therapeutic change may be beneficial to both parties.

CHALLENGE

■ Are there characteristics that are typical of professionals from different specialities?

■ List all the health and social care professions and write next to each the characteristics you would attribute to them. If you know a professional from another discipline, ask them to do the same exercise and see how your answers compare.

■ In an interprofessional group, consider which aspects of these characteristics you think are positive/negative, realistic/unrealistic. Do you personally feel you chose your profession because of such representations?

Unconscious defences: why we don't always work in a person-centred way

It was suggested in the introduction that consideration of our *selves* represented a stepping stone on the path to a realignment of services towards more person-centred and interprofessional approaches. However, if we are as inclined to distance ourselves from the nature of our working environment as we are from people's distress, then our efforts may be in vain.

Research by Menzies (1960, Menzies-Lyth 1988) identified social systems used in nursing as defences against anxiety and a way of managing stress in the workplace. This work has been supported and developed following observations made in a variety of care settings (Obholzer & Roberts 1994). These writers focus on unconscious processes in organisations, drawing on psychodynamic and systems theory. A central notion is that both individuals and organisations develop defences against difficult emotions encountered in care environments that are threatening or too painful to acknowledge. Some defences are healthy and protective in that they enable practitioners to cope with stress, fatigue and distress and to develop through their work. However, some can obstruct reality awareness and hinder the task of delivering person-centred care. Central to these defences is *denial*: pushing thoughts, feelings and experiences out of conscious awareness because they are too anxiety pro-voking. Although the authors may have interpreted these strategies as uncon-scious actions, whether deliberate or not the impact on the client is often the same. Where defence mechanisms are unconscious, they can be harder to rec-ognise and address.

Professionals may enter the clinical situation with a clear intention to prac-tise in a person-centred manner, but clinical environments can be emotionally overwhelming. Professionals may reduce the potential impact of engagement with the service user's distress by adopting conscious and unconscious strate-gies that distance them from that distress:

- Minimising the possibilities for a nurse/patient relationship with atten-tion singularly focused on tasks. It is a few short steps conceptually from unnecessarily interrupting a conversation with a client with 'Oh, is that the phone?' to 'accidentally' leaving your mobile phone switched on during a home visit to pretending to hear the phone.

- Depersonalisation and labelling: 'Mr D alcoholic, o/d, homeless ...'

- Attempts to eliminate decisions by ritualising the tasks, overstandardising procedures and routines. How many doses of medication have been missed because a patient was asleep during a drug round that was needlessly carried out at 7 a.m. or 10 p.m.?

- Scapegoating and blaming: 'Sorry your breakfast is late/cold, the night shift normally help us by getting a few people up.'

- Purposeful obscurity: fudging the issue about who is actually responsible for things; blaming staff shortages; not offering a complaints procedure.

- Reduction of the impact of responsibility by delegation to supervisors, pass-ing the buck upwards: 'I'd better ask my mentor if I'm allowed to help you.'

- Underestimation/undervaluing of personal developmental possibilities: 'a born nurse' or 'not cut out for the job'.

- Avoidance of change: 'We've tried that before and it didn't work.'

Following Menzies' framework (1960, 1988), these examples demonstrate that we adopt behaviours that are stereotypical of our professional roles as a way of distancing our inner person from the working environment. For those who would contend that it is not necessary for the practitioner to think deeply about their self as a person provided they conduct themselves professionally, it should be noted that many of those in this study will have considered that they were acting within (traditional) professional norms.

Such behaviours exploit the relationship between the institution (its rules and conventions) and the individual such that at the point of deployment the practitioner genuinely believes in what they are saying or doing. The more self-aware professional would have the option of responding more flexibly and individualistically to client need and support a service user who is at risk of feeling disempowered by health or social circumstances.

================================ **CHALLENGE** ================================

■ Have you used, or witnessed examples from your own profession of, strategies such as buck-passing or scapegoating?

■ What was the outcome and how did people respond?

Unconditional positive regard

Thus far it has been argued that how we see ourselves and how we see others are determined by a complex interaction of fixed and variable, long- and short-term, pragmatic and ideological factors, and that there are many things about ourselves and others that we can so easily be just plain wrong about. It would seem also that the way in which we communicate can reflect an underlying need to protect vulnerable aspects of ourselves. These conditions make it very difficult to for us to identify and immediately change specific aspects of ourselves and our practice. There are two responses that can support a process of continual evolution: we reflect on ourselves through tools such as the Johari Window; and we adopt a working philosophy that minimises the potential damage that might otherwise result from having fixed concepts of ourselves and others. The ability to process such knowledge of self enables us to shed new light on how we think about the person and practice in a way that frees us for autonomous, insightful practice.

The relationship between practitioner and service user is paramount if we are in any way to be effective. The quality of this relationship is a core principle of person-centred care. Person-centred theory has its roots in the work of the psychologist Carl Rogers (1902–87). Central features of Rogers' theory are that the client is *the* expert on themselves and that people:

■ Are inherently good.

■ Are motivated towards 'self-actualisation' to attain their full potential.

■ Have the capacity to grow and change.

■ Can be self-directing.

Maslow (1954) and Rogers share a humanistic stance that individuals are motivated to 'self-actualise'. However, Maslow's work postulates a human drive through his 'hierarchy of needs' from a notional space involving priorities of safety, shelter and nutritional needs, ascending towards higher-order needs of relationships, love and spirituality and culminating in 'self-actualisation'. Many texts that cite Maslow illustrate his hierarchical pyramid with the apex closed as if actualisation is something that is fully achievable at a given point in life. However, his original drawings left the apex open, inferring that self-actualisation is something that individuals need to be in quest of eternally. Rogers later developed the open-endedness of Maslow's ideology and believed that individuals are capable of 'growth' and a lifelong motivation towards their full potential, rather than being capable of exacting completion. In this respect we can see how Rogers was also influenced by Erikson's developmental theory, as he too placed emphasis on the process or journey towards something rather than focusing on the goal as an inevitable next or last step.

Erik Erikson (1902–94) was a follower of Sigmund Freud (1856–1939) to the extent that he believed Freud's ideas to be basically true, but whereas Freud argued that the development of personality began at birth and ended at age 5, Erikson felt that personality was subject to the ongoing influences of society and culture. Erikson's developmental stages encompass a range from birth through to death. Because this concept allows potentially lifelong emotional growth, it is intrinsically more consistent with a person-centred philosophy of care. Our progression through the stages of development – our journey through life – is dependent on our ability to negotiate each stage; progression is determined by our emotional success or lack of success.

Rogers' unshakable belief was that all individuals strive to achieve their 'full potential'. By way of explanation of his conviction that all humans have the ability to grow and strive to seek their full potential, he is anecdotally reported to have used the analogy of a seed potato left in the dark, damp, inhospitable environment of a coal bunker for several months. When retrieved, although the potato itself was shrivelled it bore a strong green shoot, sprouting new life.

In the case of David, above, we saw that he was brought up in a harsh and abusive environment. However, he did not perpetuate the abuse in his own family. By abusing himself only he was, metaphorically, allowing himself to 'shrivel' and risk death so that new, healthy growth might occur. Such histories are common in cases of self-harm and demonstrate how the philosophy advocated by Rogers enables professionals to re-evaluate their judgement of the service user.

The different accounts of David's experience suggest that not all the professionals knew enough about him to form this opinion. It follows from this that in the case of any service user about whom the professional might be inclined to form a negative judgement, the opposite interpretation might be more valid – hence the need for *unconditional* positive regard. Thus far this is a moral argument for positivity; pragmatically, however, practitioners are also seeking to promote the well-being of the client.

Thorne (1992: 33) explains Rogers' adversarial stance as 'given the right psychological conditions, the individual will discover both why and how he hurts ... which can lead to understanding at the highest level'. People then can begin to exhibit 'mature behaviour', a concept that Rogers defined as 'the capacity to realistically understand, take responsibility for and reflect upon one's own behaviour in relation to self and the feelings and experience of others' (Rogers 1959: 203). His notion of a fully functioning human being involves having an increasing openness to their experience and, in the case of caring for another, allows for understanding of what is happening to another without feeling overwhelmed or threatened by the experience. It is crucial, then, to listen to one's self in order to listen and be attentive in each moment, with equal interest, to the other person.

Person-centred care developed from the line of thinking that the therapeutic relationship grows from this 'unconditional positive regard' or preparedness to trust the experience of the service user rather than fear it. Sometimes it is inevitable that interventions can come into conflict with the clinical or organisational view of what is needed to aid the service user. What is being postulated here is not an either/or argument but a transferring of Rogerian thinking to modern-day health and social care. This means not letting the relationship between practitioners and organisation become more powerful than the therapeutic relationship between service user and practitioner, and remaining mindful that many service users may have fallen foul of the adverse decisions of authority figures in the past.

For example, considering the pain that David endured in order to protect his own family, one can see the traumatic effect that the revelation of the abuse of his son at nursery must have caused. Professionals working with David could not, in such circumstances, expect to call on him to trust them.

Unlike Maslow, Rogers' view of human development and the fully functioning person did not evolve from the study of emotionally healthy people but from his own clinical practice. His aspirational approach was driven by the notion that people can take responsibility for their lives and can change. This stance engendered a realistic way of thinking about and with the individual about their capacity for change. Implicit in Rogerian thinking is the belief that all people, regardless of experiences, circumstances or age, have the ability to grow – as exemplified in *Becoming a Person* (Rogers 1961). We can now begin to understand the complexity of his notion that individuals are constantly in a process of self-actualising rather than necessarily ever reaching a personal zenith of perfection in life.

In terms of the development of personality, Rogers proposed that personality is significantly shaped by the present and not entirely by childhood experiences or unconscious drives; a departure from Freudian, psychoanalytical thinking that personality is fixed in early childhood. However, Rogers stressed the importance of the mother–child relationship in its contribution to forming a person's sense of self-worth. 'Unconditional positive regard' is therefore also the phraseology he coined to describe the quality of the relationship when the child feels loved completely, unreservedly and without the need to earn that love. If the mother's love was displayed and/or perceived by the child to be 'conditional' on, for example, behaviour or achievement, then the child will internalise this and develop a sense of self that only feels worthy given certain conditions. Rogers inculcated this consideration deliberately in *how* he worked with people. Thus his person-centred approach to therapy was born out of his human development paradigm. If we are to be person centred in our work, it is crucial that we begin to reflect on how we as individuals take responsibility for our own practice and convert theories such as this into that practice. Practitioners need to centre their therapeutic relationship and be with all service users and carers in a manner that conveys equality of unconditional positive regard.

Professionals also need to reflect honestly on the principle that the service user is the expert on their experience rather than that the clinician or professional 'knows best'. Traditional models of care were previously often dominated by professional 'experts' who pathologise, categorise, label, treat and generally 'do unto the patient'. In contemporary models of care, the service user moves from a position of 'passive recipient' to 'active participant'. This is not as simple as merely keeping the service user informed of what is happening and what the clinician is thinking, but places some of the responsibility for improvement on the person. Arguably this too could be taken too literally and seen as shifting some of the blame away from the professional should treatments not be successful or completed. If a person does not comply with a treatment regime or fails to attend appointments at the prescribed time, we can too easily be dismissive and conclude that they are not engaged in the treatment, that they are non-compliant or that they are in some way deviant, and discharge them from the service that they should be grateful for. There may of course be genuine practical or emotional reasons for this; or they may be voting with their feet if we have not involved the person in any of the ways that may incorporate not just what is needed but also consideration of what that person may want.

A recent study considering patient non-compliance or adherence to medication (Jarboe 2002) revealed a stark difference between what service users said would help with compliance and what clinicians felt would help. Practitioners felt that the experience of adverse side effects, amount of medication prescribed or issues of duration and frequency would be most likely to influence non-compliance with medication, whereas these aspects were voted the least influential by service users. The latter voted that rapport and the therapeutic relationship between the service user and the clinician were the greater influencing factors for compliance (Jarboe 2002).

Conclusion

Any definition of person-centred care must accommodate the perspective of the service user. A definition in which the terms of the therapeutic relationship are specified only by the professional cannot be person centred. If professionals are to accommodate the service user's perspective, there are barriers to communication that need to be overcome. This chapter has identified that these barriers include the labels and stereotypes that we use to structure our understanding of our own, service users' and other professionals' identities.

One response to the need to overcome these barriers to communication advocated here is that professionals look within themselves for an understanding of their own values and judgements. By bringing service users into the education process, professionals have the opportunity to evaluate whether the practice that evolves from this enhanced self-awareness is responsive to their needs.

If closer collaboration between professional groups is to be attained in practice, this must be reflected in education. Interprofessional education initiatives have been developed nationally (see Milburn and Walker, Chapter 1) to address such issues, but it is likely to take time if the prevailing culture in health and social care practice is to benefit from this.

While synthesising the expert knowledge of the service user with experiential and academic perspectives in an interprofessional learning environment offers exciting possibilities for the future, the service user's perspective remains essential. Progress towards the active involvement of service users in professional education programmes is evident, but there is still some way to go before this is fully achieved. It is therefore incumbent on each professional and student actively to seek this within current educational frameworks.

References

Beresford, P., Sharmash, M., Forrest, V., Turnerand, M., & Branfield, F. (2005) Developing Social Care: Service Users' Vision for Adult Support. London: SCIE.

Byrne, P. (2001) Psychiatric stigma. British Journal of Psychiatry, 178: 281–4.

Chadwick, P. (1997) Schizophrenia: The Positive Perspective. In Search of Dignity for Schizophrenic People. London: Routledge.

Chapman, A. (2006) Johari Window, available at http://www.businessballs.com/johariwindow model.htm, accessed 29 November 2007.

Copperman, J. & Newton, P. D. (2007) Linking social work agency perspectives on interprofessional education into a school of nursing and midwifery. Journal of Interprofessional Care, 2: 141–54.

Coyle, J. & Williams, B. (2001) Valuing people as individuals: Development of an instrument through a survey of person-centredness in secondary care, Journal of Advanced Nursing. 36(3): 450–59.

Department of Health (1999) National Service Framework for Mental Health; Modern Standards and Service Models. London: Department of Health.

Department of Health (2001) National Service Framework for Older People. London: Department of Health.

Department of Health (2004) National Service Framework for Children, Young People and Care Services. London: Department of Health.

Dimbleby, R. (1947) 'More than words: An introduction to communication'. Reproduced in R. Dimbleby & G. Burton (1998) Teaching Communication. London: Routledge.

Goffman (1963) Stigma: Notes on the Management of Spoiled Identity. Harmondsworth: Penguin.

Hall, P., Weaver, L., Gravelle, D. & Thibault, H. (2007) Developing collaborative person-centred practice: A pilot project on a palliative care unit. Journal of Interprofessional Care, 21(1): 69–81.

Hayward, P. & Bright, J. A. (1997) Stigma and mental illness: A review and critique. Journal of Mental Health, 6(4): 345–54.

Herbert, C. (2005) Changing the culture: Interprofessional education for collaborative patient-centred practice in Canada. *Journal of Interprofessional Care.* May(Supplement 1): 1–4.

Hochberg, J. (1972) 'The representation of things and people. In E. H. Gombrich, M. Black & J. E. Hochberg, *Art, Perception and Reality.* Baltimore, MD: Johns Hopkins University Press.

Hornby, S. & Atkins, J. (2000) *Collaborative Care: Interprofessional, Interagency and Interpersonal,* 2nd edn. Oxford: Blackwell Scientific.

Jarboe, K. (2002) Treatment non-adherence: Causes and potential solutions. *Journal of American Psychiatric Nursing Association,* 8(4): 18–25.

Jones, A. (1999) Pathways of care in the inpatient treatment of schizophrenia: An experimental project. *Mental Health Care,* 2(6):194–7.

Kagan, K., Evans, J. & Kay, B. (1995) *A Manual of Interpersonal Skills for Nurses: An Experiential Approach.* London: Harper & Row.

Laming Report (2003) *The Victoria Climbie Inquiry: Report of an Inquiry by Lord Laming.* http://www.victoriaclimbie-inquiry.org.uk:LSTN.

Leathard, A (2003) *Interprofessional Collaboration: From Policy to Practice in Health and Social Care.* Hove: Brunner Routledge.

Lloyd, C., Sullivan, D. & Williams, P. L. (2005) Perceptions of social stigma and its effect on interpersonal relationships of young males who experience a psychotic disorder. *Australian Occupational Therapy Journal,* 52: 243–50.

Luft, J. & Ingham, H. (1955) The Johari window: A graphic model of interpersonal aware-ness. *Proceedings of the Western Training Laboratory in Group Development.* Los Angeles, CA: UCLA.

Maslow, A. H. (1954) *Motivation and Personality.* New York: Harper & Row.

Menzies, I. (1960) *A Case Study in the Functioning of Social Systems as a Defence against Anxiety.* London: Tavistock Institute of Human Relations.

Menzies-Lyth, I. (1988) *Containing Anxiety in Institutions: Selected Essays.* London: Free Association Books.

Obholzer, A. & Roberts, V. Z. (1994) *The Unconscious at Work: Individual and Organisational Stress in the Human Services.* London: Routledge.

Price, B. (2006) Exploring person-centred care. *Nursing Times,* 20(50): 49–56.

Repper, J. & Perkins, R. (2005) *Social Inclusion and Recovery: A Model for Mental Health Practice.* London: Bailliere Tindall.

Ritchie, J., Dick, D. & Lingham, R. (1994) *Report of the Inquiry into the Care and Treatment of Christopher Clunis.* London: HMSO.

Rogers, C. R. (1959) A theory of therapy, personality and interpersonal relationships. In C. R. Rogers (1977) *Carl Rogers on Personal Power.* London: Constable.

Rogers, C. R. (1961) *On Becoming a Person: A Therapist's View of Psychotherapy.* Boston: Houghton Mifflin.

Russell, S., Daly, J., Hughes, E. & Hoogs, C. (2003) Nurses and 'difficult' patients: Negotiating non-compliance. *Journal of Advanced Nursing,* 43(3): 281–7.

Sayce, L. (2000) From Psychiatric Patient to Citizen: Overcoming Discrimination and Social Inclusion. London: Macmillon.

Social Exclusion Unit (2004) *Action on Mental Health: A Guide to Promoting Social Inclusion.* London: Office of the Deputy Prime Minister, http://www.socialexclusion.gov.uk.

Summerfield, D, (2001) Does psychiatry stigmatize? *Journal of the Royal Society of Medicine.* 94: 148–9.

Thorne, B. (1992) *Carl Rogers.* London: Sage.

Winefield, H. R., Murrell, T., Clifford, J., Farmer, E. (1996) The search for reliable and valid measures of patient-centeredness. *Psychology for Health,* 11: 811–24.

Wright, D. & De Porte, P. (2000) Pull yourself together. *Update,* 2(4). London: Mental Health Foundation.

Your Rights as a Person

Jane Arnott

Questions relating to human rights encompass a complex interplay between legal and ethical frameworks. This chapter includes a brief review of the history, philosophies and key influences that have promoted the rights of individuals and is followed by an examination of contemporary developments. Such developments include the role of the United Nations on Human Rights and the introduction of the Human Rights Act (1998) in the UK. This has placed issues around the rights of the individual at the centre of the public arena and has contributed to the discourse around individual rights that has become an integral part of health and social care philosophy.

Philosophical enquiry is a very relevant activity for health and social care professionals to address, as it replaces the rigidity of 'black-and-white' reasoning with the 'grey' realities of the human experience. Seedhouse described philosophy as:

> an essential part of the way in which we understand the world. It is a process of enquiry that can have a real practical effect. The best philosophers are not happy merely to 'watch the wheels turn'. They know that what they do can help produce better wheels, or even rearrange those wheels so that a new machine is created. Philosophy can rejuvenate practice.
>
> (Seedhouse, 1995: xiv)

This chapter challenges you to:

■ Examine the concept of the rights of the individual and the challenges this presents for health and social care professionals as they seek to work with service users and communities to plan and deliver care.

- Consider the relationship between the rights of the individual and the rights, responsibilities and duties of the professional.

- Focus on the complexities this brings as practitioners seek to work within the confines of their appropriate codes of professional conduct, health and social care legislation and available resources.

The chapter is structured in a way that enables you to explore the complexities of addressing the rights of the individual and reflect on your own beliefs and values, in order to bring new understanding and learning to the workplace and, in Seedhouse's words, 'rejuvenate practice'. To assist in this process, a number of challenges are presented and you are asked to identify and examine a range of issues using the theoretical principles discussed in the chapter.

Health and social care provision has undergone a vast amount of change in the last few decades, which has been brought about by a range of factors that include advancing medical technologies, the influence of the media, social, demographic and legislative change and a shift in the public's perception, beliefs and expectations about what health and social care is and how services are provided. Parrott (2006) argues that there has been a shift away from the paternalistic perspective of health and social care delivery, where the expert decides what is best for the individual, to one where the service user is placed at the centre of service delivery, where their views, preferences and specific needs are discussed and services tailored to meet these perceived needs. This shift in focus presents enormous challenges as service providers and service user needs are balanced within finite resources, fiscal constraints and governmental targets, and competing inter- and intraprofessional priorities. There are also specific situations that require careful consideration, where the professional's duty of care has to override the rights of the individual so that an individual's or public safety is protected, for example in child protection cases or where an individual is assessed as not competent to give or refuse consent to treatment or care. These rights and duties are further examined in specific pieces of legislation such as the Children Act 2004 and the Mental Capacity Act 2005 (Brammer 2007).

CASE STUDY: SANDY

Sandy is in his 30s and is in hospital to undergo surgery. He has a learning disability and relies on his social worker and family to explain things to him and help him make decisions. Sandy has become very distressed since being admitted to hospital and is only calm when his family or social worker visits. The ward is very busy and short-staffed and you overhear the medical team discussing the possibility of giving Sandy regular sedation to calm him down. You are concerned about this decision, as you believe this may not be in his best interests and the team has not included Sandy or his family in this discussion. Later on a member of staff is seen giving Sandy some medication.

================================ **CHALLENGE** ================================

- What particular needs does Sandy have?

- Can you identify the different priorities for Sandy, his family and the social worker and medical and nursing team caring for Sandy?

- What do you think about sedating Sandy? Why do you think this?

CASE STUDY continued

Sandy has a learning disability and needs things explained to him in a clear, uncomplicated way. He finds strange situations very frightening and this causes him to become stressed and anxious. Anxiety can cause him to exhibit bizarre behaviour, which may appear distressing to onlookers.

In an attempt to reduce his anxiety, Sandy has spent time with his carers preparing for his admission to hospital and had met with some of the medical and nursing staff who would be caring for him.

================================ **CHALLENGE** ================================

- How have the above plans and actions met Sandy's needs?

- Has he been treated in manner that promotes his dignity?

- What other considerations are there for the staff and carers looking after Sandy?

CASE STUDY continued

Sandy needs to have surgery and without it will become increasingly immobile and will need to be in hospital for several days. It is important for him to feel comfortable and safe in this environment. If he becomes very distressed, he can exhibit self-harming behaviours. The surgical team is concerned that it will become increasingly difficult for Sandy to undergo surgery unless he is sedated.

================================ **CHALLENGE** ================================

- What are the important factors here?

- What are the key principles driving the surgical team's concerns?

CASE STUDY continued

Sandy did undergo surgery but had to be heavily sedated beforehand. The team who cared for him had met with the social worker, Jan, and the family over several weeks before Sandy's admission to hospital. He had been considered capable of making a decision to undergo surgery and had signed his own consent form. He needed urgent hip surgery and without this would have experienced increasing pain, immobility and loss of employment.

After surgery, Sandy was allocated a side room so that his family were able to stay with him. He was discharged home after five days with support from the community nursing team and made a good recovery.

Case study analysis

There are several key issues to consider in this case study. Sandy has learning disabilities and will have some specific needs over and above those of an individual without learning disabilities.

His social worker worked very closely with Sandy and his family and the medical and nursing team to promote his best interests. The team considers that he was treated with dignity and respect and encouraged to take a full part in making decisions about his care. Do you agree?

In 2005, the Mental Capacity Act became law (Brammer 2007), providing a structure to empower and protect individuals who are vulnerable and may find it difficult to make decisions. Sandy needed to have surgery to enable him to remain mobile and independent; however, he needed to understand what was going to happen to him to give his consent. This he was able to do; despite his learning disability it was decided that he was able to understand the concept of consent and the consequences of having or not having the operation. Nevertheless, the situation changed when he was admitted to hospital, where he became increasingly stressed and agitated by the unfamiliar people and strange surroundings. The consultant not only had a duty to Sandy, to keep him safe and ensure that he received the best care, but there was a real concern that Sandy might not have his surgery because of his distress and this had to be balanced against the consequences for him of not having the surgery. The consultant also had duties to the other patients, to keep them safe and minimise the anxiety they were experiencing because of Sandy's behaviour.

The ward was understaffed and busy and the medical and nursing teams were concerned that Sandy's distress had reached a level where immediate action was needed, and the welfare of other patients had to be balanced against those of Sandy. The decision to prescribe sedation for Sandy was based on the premise that this was in his best interests and would not restrict his basic rights. After the sedation had been given, Sandy's family and social worker were informed and Sandy's situation was reviewed to inform the management of the post-operative period.

Sandy's situation demonstrates effectively the delicate balancing act that health and social care practitioners are often presented with in trying to meet the needs and rights of one individual while also attempting to do the same universally. The roles and responsibilities of contemporary health and social care practice require practitioners to be able to scrutinise and reflect on what drives them to act in particular ways. Hendrick (2001) describes a relationship between the individual's value and belief system, 'moral intuition' and actions taken in everyday life. This 'moral intuition', however, is not sufficient to meet the unique challenges that health and social care may present. Practitioners also require an understanding of the key ethical theories or an ethical framework to enable them to reflect on their actions and deliver care that is in the best interests of the service and service user and reflects the diversity and complexity of their needs.

There are many ethical theories (see Beauchamp & Childress 2001 for extensive exploration of these), but the main ones that have informed health and social care practice are consequentialism, deotonology and, more recently, virtue ethics.

Consequentialism

Consequentialism sits in the teleological school of ethical theories. Teleological theories are those that are interested in end results. Consequentialism focuses on the outcome or consequence of an action, rather than the action itself. This means that the right or moral thing to do is that which results in the best possible outcome, 'the greatest good for the greatest number of people'. There are a number of consequentialist theories, but the best known is utilitarianism, which was developed by Jeremy Bentham (1748–1832) and built on by J. S. Mill (1806–73). Proponents of utilitarianism are less concerned with the concept of the right thing to do or the motives behind the actions than with the result of any given action. Simply put, utilitarians do not measure actions in terms of 'good' or 'bad', but how the action will affect the consequences. The more positive the outcome, the more likely it is that a particular action will be considered. This is known as the 'principle of utility'. For example, a health or social care professional may have to think about the consequences of being truthful or untruthful. A severely confused elderly person who has a poor short-term memory may become more distressed by a truthful response that her son has died each time she asks for him, rather than being told an untruth that her son will be visiting soon.

CHALLENGE

- Do you think that 'truth telling' is always the right action to take?

- What else might you have done in this situation?

- What other situations can you think about in your area of practice that might require you to think about the consequences of being truthful or untruthful?

A critical evaluation of the principle of utility raises some very important questions. How can an individual, or group of individuals, be sure that the action decided on will bring about the greatest good? The true impact of a certain action may not become apparent for many months or years, sometimes because of a lack of knowledge, information or scrutiny, or sometimes because the real motives behind the action might be hidden. History clearly demonstrates that actions that were believed to bring about the greatest good have in fact brought about significant pain and distress. One example is the development and licensing of the drugs. In the case of Thalidomide, the competition between companies and the incentive to make a profit led to the release of a drug that had not been rigorously tested. Thalidomide, which was believed to be completely atoxic, was deemed safe to use during a sensitive period of pregnancy to treat morning sickness. At the time of licensing this drug in 1957, no one knew about its potential side effects, which were associated with birth defects such as shortened limbs and malformations to the heart, bowel, gall bladder and uterus. Within four years of its introduction, it was shown that Thalidomide had severe side effects. The court case that ensued secured compensation for the victims and brought about government regulation of the development, promotion and sale of new drugs to protect the public (Abraham 2002).

Another weakness of the utilitarian perspective lies in how 'good' or 'bad' is defined. The desire to undertake an action that will bring the most 'pleasure' or 'good' to the greatness number could lead to elements of disadvantage or even acts of cruelty for some individuals, as the action depends on a definition of what is considered acceptable or unacceptable by society at any one time or what brings the greatest amount of pleasure. MacIntyre (1966), using the example of the Holocaust, takes this to an extreme, suggesting that the Nazi atrocities leading up to and during the Second World War could be deemed acceptable, because some held the belief that it was good and right to rid society of anyone who offended the purity of the race; hence the mass extermination of the Jews and other groups of people such as homosexuals and those with mental health problems or learning disabilities. This concept may appear completely incomprehensible to you from a twenty-first-century perspective that actions involving torture and mass murder are clearly wrong. This is not to say that such views are held universally, however, as reports from Iraq and other war zones can testify. MacIntyre (*ibid*.: 238) argues that if the acceptability of actions is measured in terms of the happiness or good without any clear definition about what these terms mean, then all sorts of behaviours potentially become acceptable: 'That men are happy with their lot never entails that their lot is what it ought to be. For the question can always be raised of how great the price is that is being paid for the happiness.'

There is a further difficulty with the utilitarian perspective when different views on what brings happiness are considered. The UK of the twenty-first century is a nation made up of a wide range of diverse cultural and social groups. Therefore what is considered good and acceptable in one area of society may come into conflict with the cultural and religious views of another. This, in turn, may lead an individual to consider that their rights are more important than those of another group or person. An example of this may be the 'right' to freedom of speech. Is it tenable for an individual with extreme views on race to be given a public forum to express these views? One answer may well be a clear 'no' if the consequence of granting such permission might lead to public unrest because of views that may cause serious offence. There may be legal as well as ethical consequences. A fundamental belief in the right of all people to express their views may lead to a counter argument about the freedom of the individual to be protected from extreme views that may lead to racial hatred or violence against a particular sect or religion.

Seedhouse (1995) identifies another problem with the utilitarian approach to health and social care provision. That is that in an attempt to bring about the 'greatest good for the greatest number', some individuals will always be disadvantaged, as the good gained is for the population as a whole, not for the individual. The notion of 'justice for all' is not realised, as benefits are not distributed fairly. The current reconfiguration of health and social care service provision into community and primary care settings (Department of Health 2006) has been driven by a need to bring high-quality care closer to home. This move may prove to be cheaper and more popular for the majority of people. However, for those who live on the margins of society or who are unable to register with a general practice, or who do not have a permanent address, their ability to gain from these improvements is not increased and may even be reduced.

Deontology

While consequentialists focus on the outcomes of an action, deontology places importance on the action itself and the obligation and duty to the individual, to others and to society. In the scenario described earlier in this chapter about an elderly confused woman, it was suggested that lying to her about whether her son was still alive might be acceptable in certain circumstances. A deontologist caring for the same severely confused elderly person might feel obliged always to be truthful and might believe that it is not right to lie to this person or indeed any person. The obligation to be truthful overrides the consequences of the action.

Immanuel Kant (1724–1804), the father of deontological theory, developed what he termed 'the categorical imperative', which enables individuals to identify those actions that are obligatory for all 'rational beings' and those that are not permissible. The principle relies on rational argument rather than intuition and therefore emotions and feelings do not (or should not) drive our actions. The categorical imperative is made up of three principles.

The first principle is the universal law, to treat humans as ends in themselves and to act as if you live in a kingdom of ends (not means to an end, however admirable that end might be). The universal principle or law means that for any action to be moral, the act must be in accordance with a set of rational principles, which must hold true for everyone:

> There is ... only one categorical imperative. It is: Act only according to the maxim by which you can at the same time will that it should be a universal law.
>
> (Kant 1785 cited in Bowie 2004: 58)

Therefore a principle and the subsequent action must be able to be applied universally. For Kant lying was an immoral act, because if everyone lied (universal principle) it would be difficult to determine what is true and what is false. He believed that there were no circumstances in which lying was acceptable, as lying always hurts someone or violates the law and if everybody lied, society would break down.

The second principle requires us to treat 'humans as ends in themselves' and describes the individual's duty to pursue the well-being and happiness of others. This can only be permissible if one person's happiness does not interfere with that of another.

The last of three principles requires an action to be carried out in such a way that rules apply to the individual, others and society: I must not steal as others do not steal, stealing is wrong.

CHALLENGE

■ What do you think of these principles?

■ Do you agree with them?

■ What would society be like if everyone actually operated in accordance with these principles?

The deontological perspective describes the difference between duty and what an individual might like to do. However, it does raise some difficulties for professionals working within in the health and social care setting. If the service has finite resources, then the categorical imperative cannot be implemented, as one individual will always be denied resources to allow another to receive care. It would be inappropriate to withhold services because this cannot be applied universally.

One way of regulating the distribution of health resources is through the National Institute of Clinical Excellence (www.nice.gov.uk). Look at its website and see if you can determine the ethical framework(s) that underpin its work, then answer the following questions.

CHALLENGE

■ Consider issues of resource distribution in the context of the 'postcode lottery' that operates in relation to a number of treatments.

■ How does it relate to National Institute of Clinical Excellence (NICE) guidelines?

■ Does NICE work on universal principles?

Virtue ethics

Virtue ethics theory is focused on defining 'good people' and what makes them good. Modern virtue ethics theory has grown out of the writings of the ancient Greek philosopher Aristotle, who believed that when we undertake something we have a goal in sight, and that the ultimate goal is the chief good, the greatest good. This may sound like a teleological theory (the end result justifies the means), however what is different in virtue ethics is the emphasis placed on virtues, or qualities of character such as courage, honesty and modesty. These qualities are demonstrable in the actions and choices an individual makes and are integral to the individual as a whole, not just 'skin deep'. Such qualities enable individuals to behave in a moral way and are essentials of professional behaviour.

MacIntyre (1985), the father of modern-day virtue ethics, describes a moral society where there is a consensus on common virtues and a wish to aspire to them. Virtue ethics encompass the whole of life rather than the actions we choose to or decline to take. This theory is very applicable to the professional, as the nature of health and social care itself requires professionals to be compassionate, kind, patient and courageous in order to achieve the greatest outcome. Furthermore, Bowie (2004) argues that this theory requires an individual to reflect on what drives their actions and therefore to grow in understanding of self and what it is to be human, and in turn behave in a *moral* and *virtuous* way. Raphael (1994: 79) offers an insight into the dilemmas and challenges for practitioners working within diverse ethical frameworks:

> In utility-value, when rated as means, human beings are unequal. But when we think of human beings as ends, not as means, this kind of rating does not apply. The unequal rating of men (sic) as more or less valuable depends on their efficiency, as means, in meeting the ends of other people. Valuing them as ends, as beings whose own ends (desires and choices) are to be respected, obviously does not have that kind of dependence.

Deliberations about such ethical perspectives inform and often underpin decisions made in health and social care. Practice imperatives would suggest that people may take up one position or the other in attempting to meet the needs and rights of the service user. In the real world of health and social care, professionals need to develop, as Seedhouse (1995) describes, 'a competence in ethical thinking' in order to juggle these ethical perspectives regularly as they work within codes of conduct and professional practice, establishing with service users what the best outcome is and ensuring that service users are empowered to make these decisions. All professionals are governed by codes of conduct, which describe their obligations and duties. These are underpinned by principles of doing no harm and promoting dignity, placing the client at the centre of their work and ensuring that professionals are accountable for the quality of their work and keeping their knowledge and skills up to date (British Association of Social Workers 2002; Nursing and Midwifery Council 2004). In some circumstances, professionals find themselves in situations where decisions have to be made about limited resources and an absolute duty to place every service user at the centre of decision making becomes impossible as resources are finite and one service user's rights must override another's.

The execution of sound decision making requires an examination of the relationship between societal, professional and individual value systems and how this interplay can influence the outcome for the service user, for good or ill. Adams *et al.* (2002) identify a dynamic relationship between the values of social care practitioners and the changes in society, and analyse how this process influences practice. This ability to evolve and respond to change holds for all professions, although there may be values that are specific to one area and not another or are interpreted differently because of the nature of the role. However, what is important here is to remember that whatever value differences exist between different professions, it is the individual receiving care who needs to remain central to the deliberations of the stakeholders, not the differences among them.

In the course of our non-working lives, most individuals are not confronted with life and death decisions, nor are they required to take responsibility for recommending the removal of a child from his or her parents into care. Some decisions pose huge challenges for an individual practitioner, as the duties they might be called on to perform or assist with may come into conflict with their own personal value system. A nurse, for example, who believes in protecting life may find caring for someone who has chosen not to undergo a particular medical or surgical procedure difficult to comprehend. The nurse must adhere to the patient's wishes and put his or her own beliefs to one side. This is clearly described in the NMC Code of professional code of conduct (NMC 2004), which states:

> You must respect patients' and clients' autonomy – their right to decide whether or not to undergo any health care intervention – even where a refusal may result in harm or death to themselves or a foetus.
>
> (NMC 2004, 3.2: 5)

This example raises an important question about how health and social care professionals manage the dissonance between their own value systems and those of the individuals they come across in their daily working lives. Parrott (2006) and Hendrick (2001) identify a group of values that transcend professional boundaries and have provided a secure foundation for all practice, and indeed can be traced back across the centuries. These include compassion, respect for life, promoting dignity, doing no harm and promoting justice and self-determination.

Beauchamp and Childress (2001) describe compassion as 'the active regard for another's welfare', which leads to actions that seek to alleviate suffering brought about by factors such as illness, disability, social and economic circumstances. Compassion also requires a willingness to accept another individual as they really are and to treat them with dignity and respect. Although health and social care practitioners may feel uncomfortable about a service user's decision, they can deliver care for that person in an accepting and non-judgemental way, promoting dignity and respect. Biestek (1961 cited in Thompson 2000) describes this approach as a fundamental human right and argues that it is important to separate out the acceptance of the individual and the non-acceptance of certain behaviours and actions in order to facilitate good working relationships between the professional and the individual.

The application of the values described above to everyday practice is complex and at times may appear 'tokenistic'. For example, self-determination requires an individual to have access to the right information to be able to make choices. Professionals may believe that self-determinism is a good thing; however, Tritter and McCallum (2006) argue that those who are in the most disadvantaged sections of society may be unable to engage fully in services as there is often a huge gap in understanding between those seeking services and those delivering services. Brewer *et al.* (2006) demonstrate repeatedly in their report on poverty that where the greatest social inequalities exist, there is a considerable gap between those who access education, gain employment and have greater self-determination.

CASE STUDY: SUKI AND WINSTON

Suki and Winston and their 2-year-old twin girls, Chloe and Ellie, have just moved into the area. They tell you that they have become friendly with Ian and Mandy who live nearby and have occasionally left Chloe and Ellie in their care. You know Winston and Suki and are concerned by what Mandy and Ian have told you. You consider this to be a risky situation as Ian is an alcoholic, with a history of violence and intimidating his neighbours. He has been in prison twice for causing serious criminal damage. Mandy's first child from a different relationship was taken into care. You have been working with Mandy and Ian because there have been child protection concerns for their children, Joel and Zac. A case conference had been convened recently because of these concerns and Joel and Zac were placed on the child protection register.

Suki has a long-term mental health condition and is currently receiving psychotherapy. Winston works irregular hours as a delivery driver. Suki and Winston have no family and friends nearby to help with care and they also have financial problems. Suki would like to work for a few hours when she feels better.

You arrive at Suki and Winston's house for a visit and meet Mandy and Ian, who are just leaving. They tell you that Chloe and Ellie have been with them while Suki has been at the doctor's.

CHALLENGE

- How might this chance meeting influence you?

- What are the important issues for the health and social care professionals?

- Whose rights need protecting in this scenario?

- What are the conflicts between promoting and protecting the rights of those concerned?

CASE STUDY continued

The rights of the child to be kept safe and protected from potential harm are of paramount importance in this scenario. The health and social care professional has a duty of care to the child, but Mandy and Ian also have a right to confidentiality and therefore the professional must not disclose private information about Mandy and Ian to Winston and Suki. Suki also has a right to health care and without the psychotherapy she may not be able to care for her children, as her condition may deteriorate. In the past Winston has had to give up work to care for Suki, but he is very reluctant to do this again as, in addition to the money and status he gets from work, he feels he needs some space away from Suki, as she can be quite demanding.

CHALLENGE

- What action could the health and social care professionals take to fulfil their duty to protect the children in these families and also maintain confidentiality about the couples involved?

- Does Suki have the right to psychotherapy? Does Winston have a right to work? What are the professionals' responsibilities in this situation?

- How could the health and social care professionals support Suki and Winston?

- How can the health and social care professionals support Mandy and Ian? What are their rights? What are the ethical issues involved?

CASE STUDY continued

The health visitor and social worker met with Suki and Winston to develop a supportive care package. Suki and Winston disclosed that they were not happy with the informal arrangement with Mandy and Ian. Suki did not like the way Ian spoke to Mandy and his children.

The health visitor and social worker were able to discuss the themes of these concerns without disclosing confidential information about Mandy and Ian. Suki and Winston were also involved in developing an alternative childminding plan that would allow Suki to attend her psychotherapy sessions and keep their children safe.

The family was referred to the local Sure Start and, in agreement with Suki and Winston, the following package was put into place. Chloe and Ellie were given places at the Sure Start nursery so that Suki could attend her psychotherapy sessions. The family was also invited to join in with other activities, such as parenting groups, cookery sessions and fitness classes. Suki felt that this would also help her to make new friendships.

========= **CHALLENGE** =========

▪ How will the above support package meet some of the rights of the individuals concerned?

▪ How have the practitioners involved complied with their duty of care?

CASE STUDY continued

The social worker visited Mandy and Ian and clearly outlined why it was inappropriate for them to care for Suki and Winston's children, although this had to be delivered without disclosing confidential information about Suki and Winston. Mandy and Ian asked about the Sure Start nursery, as Suki and Winston had told them about it. The social worker told Mandy and Ian that she would look into this and see if it would be possible to offer Joel and Zac places.

She also reminded Mandy and Ian that one of the decisions of the child protection conference was that they must both attend anger management sessions. If Sure Start places were found for Joel and Zac, this would mean that Mandy and Winston could attend an anger management programme. In her own mind, the practitioner felt that this would be an excellent way of monitoring the situation with Joel and Zac, although she did not share this thought with Mandy and Ian at the time.

========= **CHALLENGE** =========

▪ Are there any problems with this approach?

▪ What rights do Ian and Mandy's children have?

▪ What is the practitioners' duty to each family? Are they equal in worth?

This is a complex case scenario and describes the difficulties in working with families with a diverse range of needs. The case study demonstrates how professionals are able to work with individuals in a compassionate way that promotes dignity and respect. It also raises the question of whose rights should be given greater precedence.

The use of utilitarian and deontological theories promotes an understanding of human rights in a range of situations. Human rights are important in setting standards and emphasising the importance of fundamental values such as respecting the lives of others, dignity, confidentiality and fairness; however, they do not constitute an ethical theory. Indeed, rights-based theories are perceived to be limited and, as Beauchamp and Childress (2001) state, impoverish 'our understanding of morality, because rights cannot account for the moral significance of motives … virtues and the like'.

Human rights and professional ethics

The concept of human rights has had a long history and can be traced back as far as the fourth century BC and the Babylonians. The principles contained in such documents such as the Magna Carta (1215), the English Bill of Rights (1689), the French Declaration on the Rights of Man and Citizens (1789) and the United States Constitution and Bill of Rights (1791) laid the philosophical foundation for contemporary human rights. Thomas Paine, writing in *The Rights of Man* (1791/1991) contends that 'Rights are inherently in all inhabitants' and that the main purpose of government is 'to protect the irrefutable rights inherent to every human being'.

John Stuart Mill's model of libertarianism, which he developed during the middle of the nineteenth century, pushed the philosophy and understanding of what constitutes human rights to a new level and is generally considered to be the first generation of human rights to include the rights of women. Mill asserted that the value of freedom and autonomy depended on the context in which it was to be used. The main role of human rights was to promote freedom of choice and prevent state intervention into the freedom or 'sovereignty' of the individual, provided that the rights of that individual did not cause harm to another individual and thereby infringe the latter's human rights. Mill's theory led to further debate as the value of these rights was scrutinised. This demonstrated the conflicting opinions between his ideology and the societal values of the time.

During the late nineteenth and early twentieth centuries, Mill's theories developed further and led to a new understanding about the responsibility of the state and its role in providing a safety net to promote equality and justice for all citizens. Several pieces of legislation were introduced to replace the old political philosophy of 'laissez faire', which relieved the state of any collective responsibility for the welfare of its people with a system of benefits that took account of the needs and rights of the poorer classes in society. Health and education legislation was passed; the National Health Insurance Act of 1911 introduced sickness pay; and the right to vote was extended to all men and certain women in the Representation of the People Act (1918). The impact of the aftermath of the First World War, the General Strike of 1926 and the Depression of the 1930s culminated in the Beveridge Report of 1942, which sought to eradicate the five social evils of 'want, disease, squalor, ignorance and idleness'. There quickly followed another swathe of legislation, which included the 1944 Education Act and the inception of the National Health Service in 1948. In less than half a century Britain had become a welfare state based on collectivist or universal principles, where the welfare of its citizens was became increasingly the responsibility of the state and access to health care and education was upheld as a right for all (Alcock *et al.* 2003).

In 1945 the United Nations was established. The horrors of the Second World War placed human rights high on its agenda and 1948 saw the United Nations' Universal Declaration of Human Rights. A set of principles was created to promote and protect human rights and address the needs of the most vulnerable in society and for governments to take positive action to secure these rights. These human rights were based on the premise as described by Article 1 of the Universal Declaration that 'all human beings are born free and equal in dignity and rights. They are endowed with reason and conscience and should act towards one another in a spirit of brotherhood.' The Universal Declaration of Human Rights was applied internationally as a common standard. Many governments have incorporated its principles into national health and social care policy and legislation since 1948. The UK's Human Rights Act 1998 recognises that minimum and fundamental human rights belong to all its citizens.

Human rights and professional practice

In this context, human rights describe the relationship between the individual and the state and define what governments can and cannot do to and for individuals. They have also been divided into civil and political rights and economic, social and cultural rights. Therefore human rights range from freedom from torture, the right to vote, protection from invasion of privacy and from arbitrary arrest, to a minimum standard of what the state must provide for its people in terms of social security, shelter, food, medical care and basic education. Human rights are part of being human and therefore should apply to all.

CHALLENGE

Reports in the media sometimes suggest that the human rights of certain individuals enable them to enjoy freedoms and escape justice while victims suffer. This may raise some fundamental ethical issues for you as a person and as a professional.

■ What do you know about human rights legislation?

■ Do you think it should apply to everybody?

■ If not, who not and why not?

■ What do you think of the way it is discussed in the media?

■ Can human rights principles help you in your professional work? How?

Health and social care professionals have a duty to ensure that an individual's human rights are met and this is enshrined within codes of conduct, where rights such as confidentiality, safe and effective person-centred care are described. However, health and social care professionals also have their own rights that need to be met in order for them to carry out their daily work, and therefore the organisations and people with whom they work have a duty to ensure that professionals' rights are upheld and systems put in place to meet the needs of the workforce. Professional rights include:

■ Having the resources to undertake a role.

■ Being in a safe environment.

- Being given time to attend training and education to keep updated in order to deliver sound evidence-based practice.

One of the major themes running through government policy is the need to address social and health inequalities. Human rights legislation promotes concepts of justice, fairness and equality. Inequalities in the apportionment of resources persist and the concept of apportionment is particularly relevant to the UK health and social care agenda of the twenty-first century, where resources are finite, services are target driven and inequalities between the richest and poorest members of society are increasing (Department of Health 2006).

This raises real challenges for health and social care professionals as they seek to be fair when addressing the needs and rights of individuals. Health and social care professionals possess rights of their own and in this context are endowed by society with some moral authority to decide where rationed resources should be allocated through their professional knowledge, responsibility and accountability. Evidence from the so-called postcode lottery approach to health and social care (Department of Health 2000) would question the efficacy of this moral authority and challenge the equality of access to specific care, on the grounds of human rights. Hart's Inverse Care law (Tudor-Hart 1971 cited by Appleby & Deeming 2001) describes the relationship between need for and quality of health care. Those most in need are least likely to receive it because of income inequalities and, where the greatest health and social care needs exist, the provision and standard of services are often inferior. The fundamental human right to equitable health and social care is therefore called into question.

Health and social care practitioners also have a duty of accountability, which provides them with the authority to carry out their practice but requires that they must do it in a way that is accountable to service users, to their profession and to the general public. Caulfield (2007) highlights four ways in which professionals are accountable, or what she calls four pillars of accountability:

- Professional.

- Ethical.

- Legal.

- Employment.

These elements can provide some guidelines in determining the best way to progress in issues of complexity and uncertainty. The next case study examines the competing rights of a vulnerable individual and group of individuals and whose responsibility it is to meet those rights. The scenarios also raise issues about professional rights and ask you to consider what these rights are.

CASE STUDY: MR SINGH

It is a Saturday evening, the X-ray department is very busy and there are only two radiographers on duty. Mr Singh is 85 and fell while out buying his newspaper. He was brought into hospital by ambulance. He is brought round to the X-ray department on a trolley with a suspected fractured upper arm. The nurse reports that she cannot stay with him as the Accident and Emergency Department is short-staffed and there is a huge backlog of people waiting to be seen, so she has been told to return immediately to the department.

Mr Singh is confused and is left unaccompanied and you observe him trying to get off the trolley. This puts you in a really difficult position, as people have been waiting for a considerable time for an X-ray and are beginning to complain. However, if you leave Mr Singh on his own he might try to get off the trolley and sustain further injuries. You ring for some assistance and are told that there is no one available to help.

CHALLENGE

- What are your responsibilities to the patients that have been waiting?
- What is your responsibility to Mr Singh?
- Who has priority in this situation, Mr Singh or the queue of waiting patients? Outline the rationale for your answer.

CASE STUDY continued

Mr Singh becomes more distressed and agitated and you decide that you need to summon help. Your colleague tells you that Mr Singh is not your responsibility and you have to get on with the X-rays.

CHALLENGE

- Is your colleague acting appropriately?
- How are you attending to Mr Singh's rights?
- What action could you take to meet the rights of the waiting patients?

CASE STUDY continued

You tell your colleague that Mr Singh is too distressed to undergo an X-ray unless you get further help. You say that you will explain to the waiting patients what is happening. You are also aware that other people in the waiting area are becoming distressed by Mr Singh's situation.

You contact the Accident and Emergency department and explain your situation. The person in charge can send help. You and your colleague agree that one of you needs to attend to the waiting patients, while the other stays with Mr Singh until help comes. One waiting patient complains because he has been made to wait longer because of this situation.

CHALLENGE

■ How would you respond to the patient who complains?

■ Have you made the right decision about Mr Singh?

■ Whose rights were more important? Were you right to challenge your colleague?

This is clearly an area where complex competing needs and responsibilities will influence professional practice. Think about the rights of each individual in the situation and how professional relationships can affect people's rights.

CASE STUDY: MR AND MRS JONES

Mr and Mrs Jones have been married for 60 years and have rarely spent time apart. Mr Jones recently fell in the garden and was badly bruised. He has lost his confidence and his family are concerned that he is rapidly becoming confused and forgetful. Mrs Jones has been using a wheelchair for 10 years and relies on her husband to support her with some of the talks of daily living.

The Joneses' son and daughter would like their parents to go into care and Mr Jones becomes very distressed when this is discussed, as he is frightened of being separated from his wife. Good care provision in the area is overstretched and it is doubtful that they could be accommodated together.

CHALLENGE

■ How might this situation affect your decision making?

■ What are the issues for Mr and Mrs Jones?

■ What are the issues for their family?

■ What are the issues for the professional team involved?

CASE STUDY continued

Mr and Mrs Jones, their family and the social worker, district nurse, occupational therapist and care coordinator meet to convene a case conference. The conference considers a range of options.

Option 1

The district nurse reports that Mr Jones appears less confused recently. She feels that the painkillers he had been taking may have made him drowsy and confused. He is no longer taking these and has been able to manage most things. She reports that there is regular support from neighbours who come in twice a day.

The occupational therapist has visited Mr and Mrs Jones. She has undertaken a falls assessment and has recommended to Mr and Mrs Jones that further adaptations to the home and garden are undertaken to make the environment safer. Mr Jones has agreed to the installation of a system to raise an alarm. The occupational therapist notes that Mr Jones tires easily but does not appear confused.

The social worker has suggested that periods of respite care can be arranged to give Mr Jones a break from his caring role. The care coordinator is able to provide a continued carer service and the designated carer would like to undertake more of this for Mr and Mrs Jones.

Mr and Mrs Jones' daughter lives nearly 100 miles away and their son lives abroad, so neither is able to offer practical support. They visit infrequently and have been shocked by the deterioration in their parents' health and ability to manage. They really do not think it is reasonable for the couple to remain at home. Mr and Mrs Jones agree that they are less active and need more help to be able to manage, but are willing to receive support to help them remain independent. They clearly state that they want to stay together and do not want to go into a home.

CHALLENGE

■ What is the role of the case conference? How does it assist in meeting the rights and needs of Mr and Mrs Jones?

■ What are Mr and Mrs Jones' rights?

■ Do the family have rights? What about the daughter's beliefs?

■ How does Option 1 meet their rights?

■ What might not be met by Option 1?

CASE STUDY continued

Option 2

Mr and Mrs Jones' children express their concerns and would like to know what other options are possible. The social worker and care coordinator inform the family that it is unlikely that Mr and Mrs Jones could be accommodated in residential care together, the provision in the area is expensive and it is unlikely that Mr Jones' needs would be met in residential care.

There will be significant cost implications and Mr Jones would like to use the money to buy in help so that they can remain together in their own house rather than going into a home. Mr and Mrs Jones' daughter says that she feels that this solution is only a stopgap and the conference is avoiding the real issues. She is appalled by the state of the house and is very worried by her father's state of health.

CHALLENGE

This scenario identifies the difficulties in working with families and balancing rights, but also being sensitive to beliefs and value systems.

■ The professionals working with this family may also have to examine their own beliefs. What do they think about the daughter's reaction?

■ The daughter appears to be upset and angry about her parents' situation. Is this guilt?

■ Is it frustration or does she resent having to be responsible at such a distance?

■ What is the consequence for the agreed outcome if the individuals involved do not understand each other's perspective? How does this affect partnership working?

■ To whom are the practitioners accountable?

Conclusion

This chapter has attempted to describe the ethical complexities of health and social care practice and how practitioners need to engage in ethical discussions in order to change and improve the way in which care is delivered. Human rights in relation to health and social care provision are about the need for the respect and protection of individuals' rights and the fulfilment of these rights. The latter can only be realised if they are enshrined in law. Balancing the rights of individuals and professionals requires an understanding of the complexity of the health and social care environment and a depth of professional integrity, where the ability to empathise with and reflect on the diversity of values, beliefs and what is available drives decision making. The four case studies presented in this chapter demonstrate the need for professional integrity and identify that decisions taken with people about their lives cannot be made in a moral vacuum, but need to be within a framework that considers the individuals concerned, their rights and the duties and rights of the professionals involved.

References

Abraham, J. (2002) Making regulation responsive to commercial interests: Streamlining drug industry watchdogs. *British Medical Journal,* 325: 1164–9.

Adams, R. Dominelli, L. & Payne, M. (2002) *Social Work Themes and Issues and Critical Debates.* Basingstoke: Palgrave.

Alcock, P., Erskine, A. & May, M. (eds) (2003) *The Student's Companion to Social Policy,* 2nd edn. Oxford: Blackwell.

Appleby, J. & Deeming, C. (2001) Inverse Care Law. *Health Service Journal.* 111(5760): 37.

Beauchamp, T. & Childress, J. (2001) *Principles of Biomedical Ethics,* 5th edn. Oxford: Oxford University Press.

Biestek, F. P. (1961) *The Casework Relationship.* London: Allen & Owen.

Bowie, R. (2004) *Ethical Studies,* 2nd edn. Cheltenham: Nelson Thornes.

Brewer, M., Goodman, A. & Leicester, A. (2006) *Poverty in Britain: What Can We Learn from Household Spending?* London: Polity Press.

Brammer, A. (2007) *Social Work Law,* 2nd edn. Harlow: Pearson Education.

British Association of Social Workers (2002) *The Code of Ethics for Social Work.* Birmingham: British Association of Social Workers.

Caulfield, H. (2007) *Accountability.* Oxford: Blackwell.

Department of Health (2000) *The NHS Plan: A Plan for Investment, a Plan for Reform.* London: Department of Health

Department of Health (2006) *Tackling Health Inequalities: Status Report on Programme for Action – 2006 Update of Headline Indicators.* London: Department of Health.

Hendrick, J. (2001) *Law and Ethics in Nursing and Health Care.* Cheltenham: Nelson Thornes.

Human Rights Act (1998). London: HMSO.

Kant, I. (1785) Groundwork of the metaphysics of morals. In Bowie, R. (2004) *Ethical Studies,* 2nd edn. Cheltenham: Nelson Thorne.

MacIntyre, A. (1966) *A Short History of Ethics.* London: Routledge.

MacIntyre, A. (1985) *After Virtue: A Study in Moral Theory,* 2nd edn. London: Duckworth.

Mental Capacity Act (2005). London: HMSO.

Nursing and Midwifery Council (2004) *The NMC Code of Professional Conduct: Standards for Conduct, Performance and Ethics.* London: Nursing and Midwifery Council.

Paine, T. (1791, 1999) *Rights of Man.* New York: Dover Thrift.

Parrott, L. (2006) *Values and Ethics in Social Work Practice.* Exeter: Learning Matters.

Raphael, D. (1994) *Ethics.* Oxford: Oxford University Press.

Seedhouse, D. (1995) *Ethics: The Heart of Health Care.* Chichester: John Wiley.

Thompson, N. (2000) *Understanding Social Work.* Bristol: Palgrave.

Tritter, J. & McCallum, A. (2006) The snakes and ladders of user involvement: Moving beyond Arnstein. *Health Policy,* 76: 156–68.

Tudor-Hart, J. (1971) The inverse care law. *The Lancet,* 27 February: 405–12.

Person-Centred Care and Interprofessional Working: The Application to Practice

6

Person-Centred Primary Care and Health Promotion

Laura Gilbert and Tim Dunn

This chapter considers:

- What health promotion means for health and social care practice.

- How the work that is undertaken within the primary care setting can promote health and empower individuals and communities to improve their health.

- The different strategies that can be used for the person-centred delivery of health promotion.

- The factors that can help or hinder the delivery of person-centred health promotion.

For every individual, the knowledge required to understand the ways in which their health can be improved and serious illness prevented should be a high priority. However, for many people other stresses in their lives may mean that their health is not as high a priority as they might wish it to be. In order for health and social care professionals to consider what health and health promotion are and how health and social work practice can influence health for individuals, it is important to have some consensus of what these words mean.

There are different definitions of 'health'. One of the best known is given by the World Health Organisation (WHO), which states, 'Health is a state of complete physical, mental and social well being, not merely the absence of disease or infirmity' (World Health Organisation 1946). However, this may not be achievable for many people and it is important to consider what challenges might be associated with such a definition.

There are also several different definitions of what 'health promotion' is, with one of the most widely accepted again being the definition from the World Health Organisation (1986), which defines health promotion as 'the process of enabling people to increase control over and to improve their health'. This is one of several potential starting points that enable national and local organisations to focus on the ways in which health can be promoted, from the use of legislation to the funding of local teams and projects to tackle poor health and inequalities in health services in specific localities.

There are a number of different models of health promotion, as outlined in Table 6.1.

Many government policies published over the last decade have sought to consider and produce action plans and targets to improve the health of the nation. For instance, *Saving Lives: Our Healthier Nation* (Department of Health 1999) highlighted the responsibilities of health and social care practitioners to promote health for all and to minimise health inequalities by working in partnership with communities, the government and individuals to improve the health of each person and local communities through partnership working.

Working with individuals on a one-to-one basis enables each person to be at the centre of their care and promotes person-centred care, with holistic decision making being the paramount consideration for health and social care professionals. However, holistic decision making involves the health or social care practitioner considering the physical, emotional, spiritual, environmental, employment, education, social, medical history and family factors for each individual, which may influence the ability of that person to make decisions about their health or the health of their immediate family. Thus the practitioner takes account of all the dimensions of the 'person' and 'personhood' that were described in Chapters 2 and 3. Being able to achieve this high standard of practice requires the individual practitioner

Table 6.1   Models of health promotion.

Model	Application to health promotion
Medical model	The absence of ill health or disease is considered to be the aim of any health promotion intervention
Behaviour change model	Aims to change an individual's approach to their attitudes and behaviour in relation to their health
Educational model	Aims to provide information to enable individuals to make informed choices and decisions about their health
Client-centred approach	The aim is for clients to be treated holistically and individually, with professionals aiming to work with and empower each person to make choices and changes concerning their health
Societal change approach	Aims for changes to be introduced at a strategic level that enable a healthier lifestyle to be achieved, for example the cessation of smoking in public places

Source: Ewles & Simnett 2003; Naidoo & Wills 2002.

to have good communication, listening and verbal skills, which may take time and suitable training to develop. Being able to make holistic assessments for each person requires time for each assessment to be undertaken comprehensively, which due to workload pressures may be difficult to achieve in some circumstances, and may require additional resources such as an interpreter to enable effective communication and the delivery of essential information to take place, and thereby enable individuals to make informed decisions concerning their health and emotional and social well-being. Furthermore, for individuals to be able to make informed decisions concerning their health and any proposed treatments, housing, access to services, benefits and any other major issues, information must be delivered in a suitable format, with health and social care practitioners adequately trained to promote health and to work in partnership with their patients/clients.

The government White Paper *Our Health, Our Care, Our Say* (Department of Health 2006) sought to encourage individuals to become involved with their local health service provision and to be more actively informed and involved with personal decisions regarding their own health. Within the current proposals, General Practitioners (GPs) are able to use practice-based commissioning to commission the health services that will best meet the health care needs of their patients. In theory, this should enable the most appropriate services to be provided for local populations. For example, areas where there are large numbers of older people may require an increased range of services to meet the needs of this specific client group, such as care assistants and services to support individuals to stay in their own homes with support if they wish to do so; whereas areas with a high percentage of young people such as university towns or cities may require different services to be commissioned to meet these different health and social care needs, with the emphasis being the movement of services and care from the hospital setting to the community. In social care, the government has introduced national minimal standards with increased investment for staff training and the aim to encourage more choices for the providers of different services within the community. The intention of the White Paper is that health and social care commissioners will work together to provide services to tackle inequalities in health and social care at a local level, with a defined focus for those with ongoing needs (Department of Health 2006). This further emphasises the need for interprofessional working.

CASE STUDY: JAMES AND JOANNA

The following is an account of one family's journey involving health and social care practitioners. As you read it, think about the number of different professionals involved in the family's health and welfare.

Twins named James and Joanna were delivered to a healthy young couple by two midwives and additional medical and theatre staff. The midwives on the post-natal ward provided support and information with regard to successfully establishing breast feeding and the importance of post-natal exercises. On the tenth day, the health visitor did the first visit to the family.

When the twins were six weeks of age, they were seen by the health visitor for a developmental check. Joanna was smiling and showing that she could fix on and follow an object, but James could not demonstrate these skills. The health visitor arranged for both twins to be seen by the GP and James was then referred to a consultant paediatrician for assessment. Emotional support was provided by the maternal grandmother, who lived close by and was a good listener. The maternal grandfather helped with caring for the older grandchild and providing transport to and from appointments for the twins.

The babies then received their first immunisations. James was seen by the consultant paediatrician at the local hospital, where mild developmental delay was noted and referrals were made to the speech and language therapist and occupational therapist at the local child development centre for advice in relation to positioning, feeding and information concerning a support group, which the mother subsequently attended and found helpful. When the twins were 15 months old, the health visitor provided information for the parents with regard to the MMR (measles, mumps and rubella) vaccination and supported them in the decision-making process with regard to immunisation in the light of the conflicting publicity that the parents and extended family had read, seen and heard on the subject.

The mother was seen by the practice nurse for cervical screening. At four and half years old, the twins started in the reception class of their local primary school, where they were seen by the school nurse in the first term and had their height, weight and eyesight monitored and recorded to exclude any abnormalities. The reception class teacher provided teaching regarding dental hygiene and the twins were seen by the dental hygienist for dental screening. In the junior school, their older sister Elizabeth was bullied by some older girls in her class. Her parents sought advice from the class teacher and the head teacher, who explained the school's anti-bullying policy, which was integrated into the class by using games and circle time to encourage the children to express their feelings about life at school, as a result of which the bullying ceased. At secondary school, both James and Joanna received sexual health information as part of the national curriculum and attended a local theatre company production on sexual health, but Joanna was distressed when her best friend became pregnant at the age of 14.

At the age of 18, James was involved in a road accident on his first day of riding his new moped. The ambulance crew took him to the local Accident and Emergency department, where an X-ray taken by a diagnostic radiographer revealed a fractured femur. James's injury resulted in him having to go to theatre to have skeletal traction applied before returning to an orthopaedic ward for a six-week stay to allow the fracture to heal. In the anaesthetic room, the cheerful interaction with the operating department practitioner reduced James's fear relating to anaesthesia. Once on the ward, James became progressively withdrawn and unhappy as he was due to have started at university, and the nursing staff referred him to the occupational therapist and art therapist, who helped him to express the turbulent emotions that he was experiencing with regard to being unable to start university as planned and the frustration and disappointment of being in hospital for a prolonged period of time. The nursing staff encouraged his friends and family to visit. The physiotherapist helped James with exercise routines to regain his strength and mobility once the fracture had healed and the traction had been removed.

On discharge from hospital, James grew increasingly distant and became involved with a group of friends who introduced him to the drugs scene in the town. He was referred to a social worker and to a drug treatment centre by the GP, where he received successful treatment and ongoing support from the community psychiatric nurses once he had returned home.

The twins' mother developed breast cancer and received support through the surgery from the GP, the district nursing team, a Macmillan nursing team and the local vicar, before dying peacefully in the local hospice. The twins' father worked hard to provide a stable income for his family, but at times found it difficult to balance the conflicting needs of his employment with the changing needs of his family. He and the twins received bereavement support from a counselling service.

The twins' grandfather had a minor heart attack due to the stress he had experienced both with his family and with the demands of his job. He was seen by the occupational health nurse for advice and support regarding returning to work and reducing the stress levels that he had been experiencing.

CHALLENGE

What does health promotion mean to you?

- What opportunities for health promotion were there for the professionals involved with this family?

- How do you think that health promotion can be delivered in a person-centred way?

- What might some of the challenges be for providing health promotion to individual patients/clients?

Take five minutes to reflect on decisions you have made in relation to your own health or on behalf of your children, for example immunisation; the use of sun-tan lotion; preventive health screening such as cervical screening; or choices related to exercise or nutrition.

- What information did you receive that informed your decision?

- How did you reach the decision you made?

- Were any health or social care professionals influential in your decision-making process or in providing the necessary intervention?

Government policy published within the last eight years has sought to place health high on the political agenda, with the recognition that health promotion is essential for improving and maintaining the health of the population, to benefit individuals, their families, their community and the economy of the nation with improved productivity and fewer days taken off work due to ill health. However, there are challenges with the implementation of such policies, which involve closer collaboration with housing, education, transport, charities, health and social care, sports and recreation facilities, faith and ethnic-specific organisations, food retailers and many others to work together to enable the best health opportunities for individuals throughout the UK. For this to be achievable, funding and adequate resources need to be provided from government budgets, which in turn often have to be raised by increases in taxation.

The budgets that are allocated by the government to health and social care providers each year frequently require difficult decisions to be made as to how services are prioritised and funded. You may have read in your local newspaper or seen on the news reporting about services where funding has been reduced or withdrawn, which causes anxiety and distress to both those who have benefited from the service or care facility and the staff that have provided the service. Local petitions and lobbying of individual Members of Parliament are examples of ways in which different groups or communities can raise the profile of certain needs, both local and national, which affect the social, physical and emotional well-being of the public. Data is collected in relation to national statistics for heart disease, cancer and mental health, homelessness and drug and alcohol addiction. This assists government ministers in making decisions related to annual budgets, with specific allocations of funding being targeted at particular health and social care concerns, for example teenage pregnancy or sexual health.

This need for closer consultation and collaboration was highlighted in *Choosing Health: Making Healthy Choices Easier* (Department of Health 2004), which acknowledges that in order for individuals to make healthier choices about their dietary intake, exercise patterns and areas such as smoking, services need to be available at a local level, with support available from trained and suitably qualified staff. In this document specific health concerns were identified, which included smoking, reduction of obesity and improvement of diet and nutrition, exercise, alcohol consumption, sexual health and mental health (*ibid.*). However, the full implementation of any government proposal requires adequate funding and resources in terms of staff, training, accommodation and equipment, which can be difficult to achieve. Once a service has been started it needs to be sustained over the following months and years, with ongoing audit and evaluation to ensure the value and effectiveness of each team or service.

The government has sought to give individuals more responsibility for the decisions that we all have to make with regard to our health. *Choosing Health: Making Healthier Choices Easier* (*ibid.*) was published after consultation with the general public and looked at the collaborative working that needs to take place between the leisure industry, schools, the NHS and retailers to enable individuals to make healthier choices about their diet, leisure activities and health.

The report's three core principles exemplify interprofessional working and person-centred care:

■ *Informed choice* – the acknowledgement that individuals need to have reliable information to enable them to make informed decisions about their health, but that special responsibility will be taken by the government in relation to children, who are too young to make informed choices for themselves. The government pledged to consider the balance of rights and responsibilities in relation to behaviour that has a direct impact on health such as smoking. This approach resulted in the legislation to ban smoking in public places from July 2007.

■ *Personalisation* – services to enable individuals to make healthy choices need to be available flexibly and conveniently in all areas of the UK.

■ *Working together* – effective partnerships need to exist between local government, the NHS, business, advertisers, retailers, the voluntary sector, communities, the media, faith organisations and many others to help individuals to make health ier choices. One example of this is the restriction on the advertisement of certain brands of fast food during commercial breaks when children are watching television, as children are known to be susceptible to the powerful influence of advertising on television.

=== **CHALLENGE** ===

■ What examples of good practice have you seen in relation to health promotion?

=== **CHALLENGE** ===

One important aspect of health and health promotion concerns tobacco and smoking. The introduction of policies by the government to regulate the purchasing and use of tobacco products were aimed at improving the health of individuals and of the public as a whole in enclosed spaces (including public transport).

■ Do you think that these policies have had a positive impact on the health of the nation and on individuals?

■ Are you aware of local initiatives for helping people to modify their tobacco consumption?

■ Do you think that the government should have a role in banning smoking or is this a matter of individual choice? How did you reach your decision?

While the concept of person-centred care is not new, the emphasis on health and social care being delivered with the individual patient or client at the centre of care planning represents a move away from the more traditional medical model, where staff would decide what was best for an individual and treatment choices or plans of care would be made around those decisions.

In relation to health promotion, the debate in recent years has been whether a 'top-down' approach – where those with control and power, such as the government, local councils, primary care trusts and hospital trusts make decisions about what will be authorised and funded – is best or whether a 'bottom-up' approach – where individuals and groups decide what they need in relation to health promotion – has a greater chance of success (Ewles & Simnett 2003).

In many countries, governments make decisions at a national level in relation to interventions that promote the health of the whole population. An example of this in England was the introduction of the smoking ban in all public places and work environments. The introduction of such sweeping measures may not be valued by everyone, but the aim is to improve the health of the majority by laws that control public behaviour. There are many examples of good practice within local practices where health and social care staff have sought to implement health promotion initiatives. For example, in some areas community nurses go into pubs, working men's clubs and supermarkets to offer blood pressure and weight checks and provide individuals with the opportunity to discuss any health concerns they might have. Some areas also have health promotion mobile units, which visit supermarkets, community centres and special events to offer advice about health, personal safety and other issues that may be of concern. Sure Start teams (www.surestart.gov.uk) were created in 1999 by the Labour government in the areas identified as having the highest levels of poverty and deprivation, with the aim of improving the life chances of children from birth to 4 years of age by multi-agency partnership working between different agencies such as health, social services, housing and education, and providing accurate information on housing, parenting skills, nutrition and benefits to promote health and well-being. One major limitation of the scheme, however, is that Sure Start is not available in all areas, which therefore limits the access of many communities who could benefit from their resources.

Levels of health care and health promotion

=============================== **CHALLENGE** ===============================

- What do the terms 'primary', 'secondary' and 'tertiary' health care mean to you?

- What personal experience have you had of accessing health services, either through your local GP practice or hospital services?

- How do we all access health services when we need them?

Being able to understand the terminology that you may hear discussed is an important element of being able to understand what services might be used by your patients or clients.

Primary health care is the term used to describe health services that are delivered in the community, such as health centres, GP surgeries, opticians, dental surgeries, community nursing teams, school nurses, podiatrists, social workers and their colleagues in social services, and the many others who enable people to receive high-quality care away from a hospital. The importance of primary health care and health promotion has been known about for hundreds of years. However, the Alma Ata Declaration made at the International Conference on Primary Health Care held in the USSR in 1978 was enormously influential in bringing public health into the international arena. This conference called on all nations to take urgent action to promote and protect the health of all people. Nevertheless, 30 years on the UK still has many areas of poverty, poor housing, poor health and deprivation; the Health Secretary acknowledged in 2004 that life expectancy was eight years less for adults living in the East End of London compared to those living in Westminster. This led to the development of 'Spearhead PCTs', 88 primary care trusts in England identified from data on deprivation, mortality from cancer and heart disease to be awarded specific funding to pilot initiatives such as health trainers, enhanced smoking-cessation services and improved school nursing provision, with targets set to improve the inequalities in health in these areas by 2010 (Department of Health 2004).

For the majority of the population, their first point of contact with health practitioners will be in the community. However, with the change in working hours of most GP practices and the loss of many Saturday-morning surgeries, many patients resort to accessing their local Accident and Emergency departments for health concerns that may not require this level of medical attention. As you might be aware, this has many far-reaching implications for the public and health staff alike, in trying to provide accessible health care for all. However, with many closures and downgrading of Accident and Emergency departments in hospitals across the UK, people have to travel much further to access health care, both for emergency care and for GP out-of-hours services.

Secondary health care is hospital-based care, where either people are referred by their GP or other health care professional or they refer themselves to the Accident and Emergency department. Hospitals and trusts receive star ratings according to the level of services and waiting times that they are able to deliver within a specific time period.

Tertiary health care is where people are referred to specialist centres for services or investigations that cannot be obtained in the local area, for example specialist children's hospitals or adult patients requiring heart surgery or organ transplantation that would not be available at a district general hospital.

The three forms of preventive health care are also primary, secondary and tertiary, but each can in reality take place in any of the three levels of health care:

- *Primary health prevention* involves services and interventions that aim to preserve health and prevent the development of ill health, for example immunisation programmes for babies and children but also flu vaccination programmes for the elderly and those who have impaired health, such as those with lung disease or who have a reduced immune system after an organ transplant. Other examples are health screening programmes such as cervical screening or well men's clinics, which also aim to promote health and provide early detection and intervention for any health concerns such as high blood pressure. Primary prevention is also concerned with promoting good mental health and well-being and helping both children and adults to have positive self-esteem and self-belief (Ewles & Simnett 2003).

■ *Secondary health prevention* seeks to monitor people with a diagnosed condition and aims to prevent any complications from developing, for example diabetic clinics that aim to monitor people with diabetes closely to prevent the development of any complications such as impaired vision or high blood pressure.

■ *Tertiary health prevention* is concerned with promoting the health of people who have a health condition that cannot be cured, for example people who have had a stroke and need aids and equipment to enable them to lead as full a life as possible. Social services and housing organisations often need to work closely together to ensure that appropriate provision is made to meet the needs of each individual.

CHALLENGE

When you are next on placement or in practice, consider the health, social and housing needs of the people you meet.

■ Why is housing an issue for health and social care?

■ How have these needs been assessed and met?

■ Who has provided the funding or equipment needed?

■ How were these decisions made and how long did the process take?

■ What were the implications for the individuals concerned?

■ What might have improved the situation?

One of the challenges with health promotion can be the resources and funding to provide the services and equipment that people may require. There may be long delays between the individual assessments being undertaken by health and social care professionals and the funding becoming available for the adaptations, equipment or housing required.

More recent health policies such as *Our Health, Our Care, Our Say* (Department of Health 2006) have sought to give the public more power in the way in which local services are planned and delivered. This has included the introduction of a new service where people are given some choice as to the availability and waiting times for appointments at different hospitals, together with some choices relating to the time of appointments to enable more flexibility around other commitments in their lives.

Doing and being healthy: Putting health promotion into practice

This section of the chapter explores the factors that may help or inhibit individuals and communities from incorporating health promotion strategies into their daily lives. We have previously identified differing approaches to health promotion, including the medical model, the behaviour change model, the educational model, the social change approach and the client-centred approach. Here health promotion will be referred to as an overall description inclusive of the above models, with a focus on client centredness. The chapter has already discussed and defined health and therefore this section will focus on strategies of potential delivery of health promotion in a person-centred manner.

In exploring health promotion, we need to consider not only definitions of health and well-being but also determinants of health. That is, what are the factors that either inhibit or contribute to communities or individuals being 'healthy'? Dahlgren and Whitehead (1991) propose that determinants of health include age, gender and hereditary factors, individual lifestyle factors and social and community networks within the overarching socioeconomic, cultural and environmental conditions. Such conditions may include access to and standards of housing, employment, water and sanitation, employment and working conditions, education, agriculture and food production.

Furthermore, when considering determinants of health we also need to recognise that there are differing ways in which people may construct aspects of their health and well-being. Ewles and Simnet (2003) identify numerous constructs of health, including physical, mental, emotional, social, spiritual and societal. Throughout individual and community lives there are many variables influencing the extent to which we are able to maintain health and wellness within these constructs. Some influences on our health are at a very individual and person-specific level and may include genetic predisposition or individual values and decision making. Equally, other influences on our health and well-being are at a greater 'community' level and may include factors such as community resources, geographical location and socioeconomic circumstances. It should not be considered that either the individual or the community factors are easier to address, as each will have differing complexities that need to be taken into account.

An occupational science perspective (Zemke & Clarke 1996) on health promotion promotes the concept that human beings are essentially 'occupational' beings and that we interact with the world around us through a process of *doing* and have an innate *need* to do (Townsend 1997; Wilcock 1993). Occupations are defined as all activities in which we engage that have a meaning and a purpose and are identifiable within the society and culture in which we live (McLaughlin Gray 1997). Pierce (2003) states that each occupational experience – that is, each experience of doing – is unique and cannot be replicated exactly. The occupation of dressing in the morning will be different each day depending on purpose, mood, social factors, temporal factors and environment. The engagement in today's occupations may well be considerably different from yesterday's and therefore require a very person-centred perspective when considering how people engage in their daily lives.

Much of health promotion is about the need to 'do' in specific ways to maintain our health and well-being. We would suggest that there fewer opportunities to 'think' healthily without a change in 'doing' that will directly influence our health. Even in mental/psychological health, while we may change attitude (or thinking) towards life, life situations and stressors, we also need the opportunity to engage (do) differently to support our approach or attitude to these situations or stressors.

The manner in which we interact with our surroundings and the daily occupations that we either choose or are obligated to engage in are both influenced by our health and have an influence on our health (Wilcock 1998). If we are feeling physically well we may choose to engage in more physical activities; if we are feeling psychologically well we may engage in activities with greater enthusiasm and greater opportunity of success with a lesser concern of failure. Equally, daily occupational engagements can influence our state of health, for example we may feel much better in ourselves after cooking a meal, successfully tidying the house or going for a walk. As humans we are complex and dynamic beings engaging in equally complex and dynamic environments. We possess cognitive, physical and perceptual skills to assist us in our interaction with our surroundings. We have social, spiritual, sexual and psychological needs that may determine which occupations we choose to engage in, and roles and habits (Keilhofner 2002) that may influence when, how and why some of these occupations are conducted. For many people, adopting health promotion strategies may require a modification from the ways they currently 'do' to new ways of doing and being.

Health promotion strategies are often communicated to the general public or intended audience via the media as a need for entire populations or specific groups of people to address. In newspapers or on television there is considerable reference to, and messages about, health preservation, including ways to prevent illness, promote fitness, retain youthfulness and maintain a healthy state of mind. Such messages may be directed as primary, secondary or tertiary health considerations. Primary health promotion issues may be those that are viewed as relevant to a majority of the population, but may be expensive to manage at a secondary or tertiary level. They are often following successfully researched strategies to address the specific concern in a preventive model, for example lowering salt intake will reduce the chances of hypertension. As such, researched health promotion strategies can be argued to be largely 'accurate'. It can also be claimed that they possess a quality of trustworthiness and generalisation across a population base. However, such assumptions *may* be in conflict with the essence of a person-centred approach. To be person centred one must consider the individual(s) within the community and negotiate priorities and strategies for maintaining or increasing the health of those individual(s) with reference to their specific beliefs, environments and lifestyles. It is possible that these negotiated actions and targets *may* reflect the overall health promotion needs and direction of the community, but that is neither a certainty nor a necessity.

To promote the health of a population within communities, we need to consider aspects such as demographics, economy, community resources (and access to these resources), infrastructures, education and the shared needs of the majority of a given population. Health promotion needs then to be refined to address the target population on the issues that are significant to that group of people. Such an approach allows a greater opportunity for focused health promotion towards a specific and recognised group. Such strategies may be global ('macro'), such as consideration of health needs of differing countries that may have quite differing constructs and determinants of health. This may also be accurate at a national level in considering the needs of one town/community in comparison to another. To promote health from a 'micro' perspective, we need to assess and consider the uniqueness of the individual(s) in conjunction with the research and successfulness of specific and possibly prescribed strategies.

For many, addressing areas of improving their health and reducing the risk of illness, disease, disability or death will require a change in either attitude and behaviour or both. As described by Keilhofner (2002), our patterns of 'behaviour' – that is, the daily activities in which we engage – are consequence of contextual factors such as space, time and sociocultural meaning and the subjective factors of our own values, interests and attractions. These factors will either consciously or subconsciously influence how and why we partake in occupations and engage in our surroundings. While many people may have the motivation to change their perspectives on health and health promotion, this must be supported by contextual factors in order to promote and sustain identified strategies of health promotion.

This is not to suggest that large-scale health promotion strategies are either unrealistic or unnecessary. However, it does take into consideration that the 'requirements' – that is, behaviours and resources of global or national directives – may at times be difficult for individuals to meet regardless of levels of motivation. Indeed, it may be argued that for some people knowing that they should be aspiring to a target that is 'beyond reach' may have the adverse effect of increasing stress, decreasing life satisfaction and sense of well-being, thus adding to the possibilities of ill health and disease.

CHALLENGE

Consider the following areas that have recently been identified as primary and secondary considerations for health promotion and education (you may be able to add to this list):

- Smoking cessation.

- Obesity.

- Stress reduction.

- Lower salt.

- Alcohol awareness.

- Regular exercise.

- Sex education.

- Immunisation.

- Calcium intake and bone density.

- Water intake.

Answer the following questions:

- Which of these areas is currently most important to you?

- Why is this important to you?

- Which of these do you currently address?

- If you do address any of these, is it as often or thoroughly as you would like?

- Are the areas of health promotion that you currently address in correlation with those that are most important to you?

- What activities do you do that address your most important area of health promotion?

- What are factors that assist you in you in addressing these concerns?

- What are factors that hinder you in addressing these concerns?

- Is it possible or necessary to address all of these concerns?

- How much would your current life need to change to address all of these concerns?

- Would your priority for these areas of health change over time?

- If yes, why?

In responding to the above challenge you may have identified various views and priorities. There will be differing perceptions of risk associated with an activity, therefore differing levels of priority given to the identified health concerns. Some of these areas will be regularly addressed within your current daily routine and others will not. You may also have identified areas of health that you hold as important yet that are difficult to address and are therefore not given the desired level of attention.

Variables that influence responses to health promotion strategies

Using the example of weight reduction as a health promotion target, let us explore some of the possible variables influencing how individuals or communities may or may not be able or wish to prioritise it as a key health concern to address. These variables are the environment, roles/identity, occupational structure, interests and attractions.

Environment

The environment in which we live can be viewed in relation to the 'micro' environment, such as immediate home, work or community surroundings, and the 'macro' environment, the wider community, social and political context. For the purpose of this discussion we will consider both micro and macro elements of the environment in relation to physical, social, cultural and political perspectives.

Physical

The physical environment encompasses both the natural and built environment. We need to consider the spaces that we have to utilise, such as our homes, neighbourhood and towns, and the equipment or resources within these spaces, for example personal equipment such as a bicycle or a community resource such as a gymnasium. If we take the example of weight reduction as a health promotion concern, then we may look at the need for individuals and communities not only to reduce or modify nutritional intake, but also to have and use opportunities to increase physical exercise. First, let us consider the requirement to modify nutritional intake. What is the range and availability of food items in the local community? Is there ready and easy access to foods that are low in fat and higher in nutritional value? Are these foods expensive? Are there a considerable number of fast-food outlets or restaurants in the area? Do these eating facilities offer healthy options? If and/or when people are able to obtain the recommended food groups, do they have the facility in their homes to prepare these foods? What are the cultural and ethnic considerations that may affect individuals' choices in these areas?

If we then consider options for increased physical activity, we need to explore the requirements of space and equipment to do so. Are there local walkways or parks? Are these considered safe? Are they lit for evening use? Are cycle tracks provided? What is the cost and availability of gym membership and what is the physical environment of these gyms like? For example, many people may be put off by numerous mirrors! Do people need or have access to specific clothing or equipment and have means of purchasing or regularly laundering such items if required?

CHALLENGE

■ Consider your own natural or built environment and the equipment/resources within it.

■ What possibilities for nutritional change and exercise are there?

Social

The social environment encompasses those around us with whom we share our lives and environments. Our social environment is likely to be a changing dynamic as we mature and develop differing roles and responsibilities and possibly live or work in differing geographical locations. Again, if considering weight reduction (exercise and nutritional intake) we need to explore the social arena of the individual(s) concerned. Constructs of our social world may be influenced by factors such as our immediate family grouping, friends and neighbours or the overall local community, socioeconomic status and employment/productivity opportunities. Some may seek opportunities for socialising within given occupations while others may seek greater solitude. The influence of the social environment may fluctuate considerably depending on aspects such as age, gender, culture, ethnicity, membership (clubs/hobbies), kinship, parental presence and the influence of other role models locally and in the media. If we were to promote exercise and nutrition to teenage boys, this would need to be with clear consideration of their social circle, both their friends and family. We would need to consider what is accepted by the boys, what is 'cool' or fashionable, age appropriate and fits with the social movements and occupations that the boys will engage in.

CHALLENGE

■ What are some of the social influences in your life that may have an impact on health promotion strategies or opportunities for you?

Cultural

While there may be clearly researched reasons for weight reduction to help achieve physical well-being and health, we may also need to consider how obesity itself is viewed in different cultures and how accepted the recommended strategies are. Some cultures may view obesity as an indication of status. Reasons for this may be the role that food plays within these communities and the associated meanings of gift giving, welcoming and hospitality. Therefore equal consideration may need to be given to the types of food used and accepted within the culture and the cooking/preparation methods employed, rather than solely how the food is used. Further to this, the opportunities and cultural attitudes/acceptance of differing exercise need to be considered.

Furthermore, defining culture purely by ethnicity is restrictive and incomplete. Many people may have a culture defined by geography, local community or perhaps family. They may be of a specific ethnicity yet live in a community or geographical area that depicts or dictates a different cultural influence.

Cultural considerations need to examine both the recommended primary (preventive) and secondary (management) strategies to ensure that these are able to be culturally accepted and applied. What is the place of increased exercise within the culture? Is this accessible to both men and women? What form of clothing needs to be worn? Does the culture value and allow time for pursuits that may be viewed as leisure or personal maintenance over productivity and community contribution?

================================ **CHALLENGE** ================================

▪ Consider the cultural influences in your current environment and the differing values and role that food and/or exercise may have within these cultures.

▪ Explore the relationship in your environment between cultural influences and issues such as drug and alcohol use.

Political

The political environment includes current government agendas, legislation and direction. Some of these have been outlined previously in the chapter. There will be many and numerous policies and legislative directives within communities that are forwarded as either guidelines or indeed legal requirements. These may range from local (community) policy and bylaws to national legislative directives. Different political parties may have varying values and beliefs concerning health and welfare. Both the financial and human cost of health and social care will be significant factors in promoting political change and direction.

================================ **CHALLENGE** ================================

▪ What are some of the current political factors that may influence your own attitudes and behaviours towards health promotion?

Values

As previously identified, health is a multifaceted concept including physical, mental, emotional, social, sexual and spiritual dimensions. For many the aim of the promotion of optimal health across all of these dimensions will be very difficult (if not impossible) to obtain. Each individual needs to make decisions regarding their own health and possibly the health of those they have direct responsibility for, for instance the parents of young children. The process of decision making may be complex, requiring the assessment of differing risk factors against what we may perceive as important or essential in our lives. Individual value systems will be significant in deciding which health promotion information or strategy is accommodated. Some of us may prioritise happiness and mental well-being over some of the more conventional perspectives of physical health and therefore our focus will be on activities and behaviours that first promote psychological rather than physical well-being. Others may have firm values surrounding physical health and maintenance of physical fitness, with the aim of reduced physical disease or ill health. Individual values are not essentially static and may change over our lifetime. The values that we hold may be influenced by culture, family or environment and will therefore change as these influencing factors change.

━━━━━━━━━━━━━━━━━━━━━━━━ **CHALLENGE** ━━━━━━━━━━━━━━━━━━━━━━━━

■ What values do you currently have that influence your choices over your own health?

■ Have these changed over time and/or do you think they will change?

■ What has influenced these changes in your values?

Roles/identity

We fulfil numerous roles during our lifetimes and have differing identities associated with these roles. Roles and identity can be both internal and external; that is, those that you perceive yourself as fulfilling and those that others view you as being. Our roles and identity may be defined by family or social structure such as father, mother, brother, sister or neighbour, or may be defined by occupation such as nurse, butcher or mechanic. Each role or individual identity may have behaviours or values that are associated with it either internally or externally and therefore have an impact on the health promotion constructs that we are either inclined towards or expected to be inclined towards by those around us.

━━━━━━━━━━━━━━━━━━━━━━━━ **CHALLENGE** ━━━━━━━━━━━━━━━━━━━━━━━━

■ Can you think of roles that you fulfil that influence your decisions about or others' perceptions of your health and well-being?

Occupational structure, habits and opportunity

This is the concept of how our daily occupations link together, the notion that one occupation may or will provide opportunity and structure for others to occur. Using the example of increasing physical activity, we need to consider where in the day such opportunities may be available and to which occupations they may be directly linked. Some of these may be formal segments of time set aside for specific engagement, such as attending a gym, while others will be more discreet opportunities enfolded within other occupations such as walking or cycling to work rather than driving.

Rarely will an occupational engagement occur in isolation to the daily or weekly occupational structure around us. For many of us, occupations have a specific temporal orientation of when and how long they occur and are therefore developed in relation to other occupations that support this. Others have a specific spatial requirement for where they occur and are therefore structured around environments that support that. The possibility and extent of structuring or restructuring of occupational engagement will be a very individual process and may require some challenging of established habits and routines regarding when, where and how we currently participate in occupations in the context of spatial, temporal and social dimensions.

- How is your day or week currently structured?

- What factors have influenced this?

- Which occupations do you have that link to or rely on others?

- How able are you to alter this routine or structure?

Interests and attractions

As discussed by Keilhofner (2002), each of us will have differing interests and attraction to various forms of occupation or 'doing'. To assist people to engage in healthy occupations, we need to be aware of what these interests or attractions are. These may be linked to our values, roles, habits or identity and/or past and present experiences. For many, the opportunity to exercise may take many different forms, each with a differing level of attraction. While we may have an interest in something, the actual overall attraction of taking part may be a lesser priority when considered against other occupational opportunities. For this reason, it is important to explore options fully, allowing people informed choices and decision making in the process of addressing health needs.

- If you were to increase your daily amount of exercise, which occupations would you choose for this?

- Why would you choose these options?

Figure 6.1 shows a model of how the different levels of person-centred health promotion referred to above are influenced by the different variables.

Conclusion

Proactive health care and health promotion are believed to be effective in reducing the incidence of ill health. However, health promotion is not only about the prevention of disease or disability When considering health promotion, we need to be able to think of the primary health strategies aimed at reducing the incidence and onset of conditions; the secondary health strategies aimed at managing and reducing the chance of reoccurrence of ill health or disease as it has been experienced; and the tertiary health strategies for managing conditions that have become established, longer term or chronic in either individuals or populations. With current established and widely accepted knowledge of the correlation between specific behaviours and habits and the risks of ill health, there can be a perception that those who then develop largely 'preventable' diseases are indeed at fault or 'to blame'. Many conditions of disease or ill health have

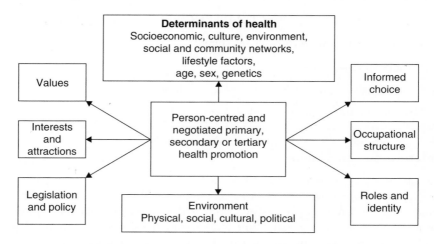

Figure 6.1 Levels of person-centred health promotion.

relatively established and accepted processes of cause and effect (this may be based on medical models, cultural beliefs or spiritual values). As we may be able to 'explain' the reasons for much ill health, this promotes the opportunity to 'blame' individuals for not paying greater attention to the maintenance of their own health through choice and/or personal responsibility. Such a blame mentality and culture have the assumption that the strategies for promoting health and preventing illness are largely and/or easily accessible; that is, able to be adhered to by the targeted population and the individuals within that population.

To consider health promotion in a truly person-centred manner is to acknowledge the concept that health promotion strategies may not always be as easy to adopt as some of the media information may have us believe. We need to consider the person's own definitions of health, values of health and health priorities; all variables that may indeed change over time.

References

Dahlgren, G. & Whitehead, M. (1991) *Policies and Strategies to Promote Social Equity in Health*, Stockholm: Institute of Futures Studies.

Department of Health (1999) *Saving Lives: Our Healthier Nation*. London: Department of Health.

Department of Health (2004) *Choosing Health: Making Healthy Choices Easier*, London: Department of Health.

Department of Health (2006) *Our Health, Our Care, Our Say*, London: Department of Health.

Ewles, L. & Simnett, I. (2003) *Promoting Health: A Practical Guide*, 5th edn. Edinburgh: Bailliere Tindall.

Kielhofner, G. (2002) *Model of Human Occupation*, 3rd edn. Baltimore, MD: Lippincott, Williams & Wilkins.

McLaughlin Gray, J. (1997) Application of the phenomenological method to the concept of occupation. *Journal of Occupational Science: Australia*, 4(1): 5–17.

Naidoo, J. & Wills. J. (2002) *Health Promotion: Foundations for Practice*, 2nd edn. Edinburgh: Bailliere Tindall.

Pierce, D. (2003). *Occupation by Design: Building Therapeutic Power.* Philadephia, PA: F. A. Davies.

Townsend, E. (ed.) (1997) *Enabling Occupation: An Occupational Therapy Perspective.* Ottawa, Ontario: CAOT Publications.

Wilcock, A. (1993) A theory of the human need for occupation. *Journal of Occupational Science: Australia,* 1(1): 17–24.

Wilcock, A. (1998). *An Occupational Perspective of Health.* Thorofare, NJ: Slack.

World Health Organisation (1946) *Constitution: Basic Documents.* Geneva: World Health Organisation.

World Health Organisation (1986) *The Move Towards a New Public Health: Ottawa Charter for Health Promotion*, First International Conference on Health Promotion, Ottawa, Nov 17–21. Ottawa: World Health Organisation/Health and Welfare Canada/Canadian Association for Public Health).

Zemke, R. & Clarke, F. (1996) *Occupational Science: The Evolving Discipline.* Philadelphia, PA: F. A. Davis.

7

A Person-Centred Approach to Safeguarding Vulnerable Adults

Georgina Koubel

All too often there is a risk that adult protection – now reconstructed as safeguarding adults (Association of Directors of Social Services 2005) – can become a procedural and administrative process, a maze of professional conflicts and competing rationalities within which the experience and perspective of the individual person at the heart of the process become obscured by the responsibilities and anxieties of the professionals working on the 'case'.

This chapter explores:

- Attitudes and values in adult protection/safeguarding.

- Who is a vulnerable adult? What makes people vulnerable?

- What is abuse? What are the signs and symptoms?

- How does abuse come to light and what legal and ethical issues should be considered in response to safeguarding adults?

- How can a social model of disability help maintain an empowering person-centred perspective and promote appropriate interprofessional working in relation to developing effective practice in safeguarding vulnerable adults?

- What are the differences and similarities between child and adult protection? What lessons can we learn from child protection?

From the shock of the Maria Colwell report in 1974, which alerted the world to the horrors of child abuse, through to changes in polices that were developed following the death of Victoria Climbie in 2001, lessons are continually being learned in the arena of child protection. These have led to the setting up of multi-agency child protection committees, the Every Child Matters agenda (2004) and the Department of Health Framework for Assessment (Jowitt & McLoughlin 2005). While there are issues that are specific to children, some of the findings are highly relevant to safeguarding vulnerable adults. The factors that seem to return repeatedly in the aftermath of these tragedies is their demonstration of the propensity for practitioners from diverse disciplines to work within their own frameworks rather than focusing on interprofessional collaboration, and the ways in which situations could have been addressed differently had they been viewed from person-centred perspectives.

The change in focus from procedure-led to person-centred perspectives would:

- Encourage the development of good communication between professionals, with clear delineation of roles and responsibilities.

- Enable all professionals to work together to ensure that there is direct work with the individual concerned that all parties are able to support.

On occasions, joint working and support can help immensely in areas where practitioners are anxious or uncertain about the nature of the tasks they need to carry out. However, as Warren (2007: 85) emphasises, working together as professionals to ensure that service users and carers are genuinely involved in participating in the processes that concern them 'takes time and emotional energy'. It is too easy for busy and anxious professionals to rely on policies and procedures and communicating (more or less effectively) with each other, leaving the service user and carer on the outside of the interaction. For a number of reasons, some of them valid such as a vulnerable individual's level of anxiety or inability to understand what is going on, it is still not uncommon for service users and carers to be excluded from strategy meetings and case conferences, despite the fact that the decisions professionals are making may have a significant impact on the lives of the persons concerned. It is important that when such meetings take place the individuals most concerned are included in the discussion, unless there are compelling reasons not to do so. To exclude someone simply on the grounds of their age, for example, is clearly unreasonable (Crawford & Walker 2003).

Elder abuse and risk in relation to vulnerable adults (Kelmshall & Pritchard 1997) has begun to attract attention over the past 15 years and it is increasingly seen that 'responding to abuse is a further important part of social work with adults' (Adams *et al.* 2002: 302). Although far from occupying the central place held in the public consciousness by the safeguarding of children, there is increasing awareness that there are also some vulnerable adults who may need protecting in a similar way. These may include people with physical or learning disabilities, those with mental health needs and those who are older, frail or lacking capacity. Within a person-centred perspective it may also be valid to look at other adults who may be vulnerable for social reasons as well as because they suffer from a particular condition or illness.

People who are perceived as vulnerable may be abused by others who come from a range of backgrounds. This may include people abused by family members or informal carers, by carers who are employed to come and provide services, or by medical, day care or residential care staff, or less frequently by strangers. Issues of power, risk and vulnerability are therefore critical to our understanding of how professionals work with issues of safeguarding adults who use services (Martin 2007). Because of their physical and emotional dependence, and at times their intellectual limitations, adults who are vulnerable are often seen as unreliable witnesses, making prosecutions against those who have abused older people or exploited those with learning or physical disabilities extremely rare (Johns 2005).

Maintaining a person-centred perspective in the face of legal and procedural processes requires an awareness of, and commitment to, person-centred values within a clear understanding of the roles and accountabilities of relevant professional personnel. The definitive Department of Health document on adult protection, *No Secrets* (Department of Health 2000), which lays great emphasis on prevention and multi-agency working, defines adult abuse in this way:

> Abuse may consist of a single act or repeated acts. It may be physical, verbal or psychological. It may be an act of neglect or an omission to act, or it may occur when a vulnerable person is persuaded into a financial or sexual transaction to which he or she has not consented or cannot consent. Abuse can occur in any relationship and may result in significant harm to, or exploitation of, the person subjected to it.
> (Department of Health 2000 in Brammer 2007: 526)

==================== **CHALLENGE** ====================

Throughout this book we have highlighted the ways in which we construct the world and its relationships through the words and images we use. Think about the kind of language we use in relation to adults who may need or use services. What do the words below mean to you? How do they define the image you have of the person who may need help or who may be abused?

■ Vulnerability.

■ Disability.

■ Frailty.

■ Invalidity.

■ Incapacity.

■ Abused.

■ Protected.

■ Safeguarded.

Why do you think there has been a move away from the concept of protection to one of safeguarding? What difference does the language make in your thinking about how to address issues around safeguarding vulnerable adults?

Powers and duties in respect of vulnerable adults

Unlike child protection where the legal framework is brought together under unified legislation, legal remedy in relation to adults is much more dispersed. There are a range of legal powers and duties available to help professionals think through their options in cases of adults being abused. Some of these are contained in criminal law while others, such as the Court of Protection and power of attorney, help deal with the financial aspects of people who need assistance. The Sexual Offences Act 2004 and the Care Standards Act 2004 may offer practice guidance. Laws relating to the assessment and provision of services, such as the National Assistance Act 1948, the NHS and Community Care Act 1990 and the Chronically Sick and Disabled Persons Act 1970, may also be of assistance (Mandelstam 1999).

The National Assistance Act 1948 gives local authorities the power to promote the welfare of people who are:

> aged 18 or over who are blind, deaf, or dumb or who suffer from mental disorder of any description and other persons who are permanently and substantially handicapped by illness, injury or congenital deformity or other such disabilities as may be prescribed.
>
> (National Assistance Act s29i)

=== **CHALLENGE** ===

If you were not too sure before about the ways in which language can frame the image we have of older or disabled people, look at the language used above.

- What does it say about the values of the time?

- How do you think concepts have changed since the 1940s in relation to older people and people with disabilities?

- How does the language we use now reflect these changes?

One of the ways in which we can start to address the negative stereotypes that are held about people with disabilities, whether young or older people, is to become aware of the ways in which these members of the community can experience discrimination.

> The characteristics of many adult service users make them especially vulnerable to discrimination and an awareness of the relevance of anti discriminatory law can help to promote good practice in this area.
>
> (Brammer 2007: 435)

=== **CHALLENGE** ===

- How do you understand the connection between language and discrimination?

- Can you think of a time when you have used discriminatory language about someone who is disabled or about an older person or an individual with a mental or physical illness?

The use of discriminatory language may not be seen as a negative perception – perhaps you felt you were being kind, making excuses for their behaviour or being overprotective. These well-meaning attitudes can sometimes hamper people's choices, rights and struggles for independence by restricting their opportunities and ignoring their wishes. While families, carers or professionals may feel that they are doing what is best for someone and intervening in areas that may lead to increased levels of risk or unwise choices, the individual may not see things as you do. Service user and carer participation in the development of services can enhance the work of professionals in exploring these dilemmas and find ways to address them (Warren 2007).

> Professionals have been perceived by clients and sociologists alike as controlling, distant, privileged, self-interested, domineering and the gatekeepers of scarce resources.
>
> (Swain *et al.* 2005)

=== **CHALLENGE** ===

■ Can you identify how an awareness of issues of power and their relationship with person-centred care and interprofessional working, as discussed throughout this book, is essential when considering the safeguarding of vulnerable adults?

Safeguarding adults

Most people are familiar with the idea that there are some children who need the protection of social services in situations where they are being abused or exploited. Unfortunately, the public perception of such situations, usually gleaned from media coverage, is that as often as not social workers have either been negligent in their duty and allowed a tragedy to occur, or have been overzealous in removing children from a home where abuse has not in fact taken place (Parton 2006). Despite the fact that the general public may only become aware of the whole system of protection when a tragedy hits the headlines, it would be fair to presume that most people accept that there are times when children do need to be protected from abuse, and that on occasion this may involve their removal from their parents or carers. Since the Maria Colwell case in 1974, there has been a series of tragedies that have had the effect of making professionals and the general public aware of the risk of abuse to children and young people. There are also considerable issues of concern in relation to disadvantage and discrimination of children who are 'looked after' by the local authority, or disabled children whose needs as children may be overlooked as professionals focus on the issues of their disabilities (Jowitt & McLoughlin 2005). There is emphasis in government policy in Every Child Matters on both person-centred perspectives and the importance of joined-up working between professionals, particularly between education and social services, which has led to changes in the way in which services are structured for children and families.

Less recognised is the role of social services, and other professionals, in the protection or safeguarding of adults. There are some similarities with the questions and dilemmas that arise in the field of safeguarding children, but there are also some very important differences. While children are seen as innately vulnerable, because of their age, size and relationships with those who have care and control of them, the parameters around which adults may or may not require assistance or protection, and the limits of statutory intervention, are much more difficult to define.

CHALLENGE

- How would you define a vulnerable adult?

- What makes adults vulnerable?

The following is the definition of 'vulnerable adult' that was included in the Law Commission work on the Mental Incapacity Act; it is significant that this term has been included recently in statutory form in the Care Standards Act 2000 (s.80):

- An adult to whom accommodation and nursing or personal care are provided in a care home.

- An adult to whom personal care is provided in their own home under arrangements with a domiciliary care agency.

- An adult to whom prescribed services are provided by an independent hospital, clinic, medical agency or NHS body (Brammer 2007: 418).

CHALLENGE

- What do you think of this definition?

- How does it help you to understand the role and responsibilities of professionals in relation to safeguarding vulnerable adults?

The model of community care actively promotes the notions of choice and independence for people who would have previously been expected to spend all or part of their lives in institutional settings, with little control over the factors that would influence their lives on a daily basis. However, this emphasis on the preference for adults who may be seen as vulnerable to live in the community also carries with it a tension between the rights and wishes of the individual and the fears and concerns of those around them for the level of risk that this may sometimes entail (Thompson & Thompson 2005).

The need to safeguard vulnerable adults does not, however, only affect those who live in their own homes. Older people and people with disabilities in residential care may often be those who are among the most vulnerable in our community. The modernisation agenda in social services (Adams *et al.* 2002) has vastly increased the involvement of the private sector in the provision of domiciliary and residential care. This raises particular issues for the safeguarding of vulnerable adults and the interprofessional, interagency aspects of adult protection, involving the setting up of the Commission for Social Care Inspection (CSCI) as an independent, overarching body to inspect private homes.

A social model of vulnerability

As with the social model of disability, where the reasons someone is unable to function effectively in society are attributed to the physical environment and the attitudinal barriers that restrict their progress (Oliver & Sapey 2006), it is possible to construct vulnerability in the same way. So while some people may be vulnerable because of something that is inherent to them – impairment, communication difficulties, mental health problems or dementia, for example – the things that relate to vulnerability may equally be problems connected with their situation or environment. This changes the emphasis within person-centred care from a model where the individual is required to change or adapt to one where it is social structures and systems that need to be challenged and to be subject to change.

For example, Michael has cerebral palsy and has very restricted mobility in his legs. As a wheelchair user he may be an active member of the community, do his own shopping and cooking, have a wide circle of friends, go to work and manage his own finances. He may be married, have children and travel abroad regularly.

Alternatively, Ralph, a man of the same age and also with cerebral palsy, may live at home with his ageing parents in unsuitable, rundown accommodation, receive minimal state benefits, rarely go out and have a very limited range of relationships.

These variations may have very little or nothing to do with the actual physical impairments that Michael and Ralph have in common.

=== **CHALLENGE** ===

■ What sorts of things do you think would have contributed to the differences between Michael and Ralph's experiences?

■ Which one do you think is more likely to be vulnerable to abuse?

So a picture is beginning to emerge of the reasons some adults may be more vulnerable than others. Many factors may contribute to the social context of the person's situation, and it is becoming clear that these issues may not always be related to the disability or impairment that the individual is experiencing.

=== **CHALLENGE** ===

Reflecting on the issues that have been discussed so far:

■ What kinds of adults may need to be safeguarded?

■ Why would they need to be safeguarded?

- Who should be responsible for safeguarding adults?
- How is this related to the concept of person-centred care?

By taking the social model of disability (or vulnerability), we are not so much focusing on what a person cannot do for themselves as looking at what can be done within the environment of that individual to help them to achieve what they want (Martin 2007). This approach requires anyone from the inter-professional team who encounters someone who may be perceived as vulnerable to take a step back and consider the social factors that may be causing their difficulties, rather than laying them at the door of the individual's age or impairment. Once the initial crisis of safeguarding one or more individuals has been addressed, time should be made to consider how to build on their strengths and abilities and what kind of safeguarding plan could contribute to supporting them to achieve the goals they want to achieve. This is the difference between 'working with' an individual rather than, however well meaningly, 'doing to' them.

It is about seeing the individual as the one who determines what they want to achieve and the team trying to find ways to get them there. It is not about being able to do everything yourself – none of us can do that – but about ensuring that the individual sits at the centre of whatever plan is devised to safeguard and support them, rather than employing a safe, systematic response that protects the organisation. Practitioners need additionally to go on to consider the possibilities for learning, empowerment and developing potential from which the individual could benefit.

The tendency to take over and do what professionals think is in the best interests of a vulnerable person is particularly prevalent in working with older people, whether they actually have the capacity to make their own decisions or whether that capacity is compromised in some way:

> We should not rely on stereotypes of dependency but, rather, actually take the trouble to work out in each situation we deal with how much or how little assistance an older person needs. Simply equating old age with dependency, with all the disempowerment this entails, is clearly not acceptable.
>
> (Thompson 2007: 78)

This, of course, is all very well in theory. However, if we look at the level of need of some individuals, and particularly at the levels of risk that may be involved, the question of how to safeguard an individual without breaching their personal wishes or human rights provides us with a range of dilemmas. In these situations, it is worth asking whether the solution or outcome that people feel would be most appropriate would be the same were the person younger or able-bodied. Is there any sense in which the person is being discriminated against because of their age or disability?

CASE STUDY: ELSIE PRICE

Take the situation of Elsie Price. Elsie, who is 85 years old, has lived on her own since her husband died six years ago. She gets some help from her son, Eric, who, following his divorce six months ago, has moved in to live with his mother. He is unemployed. Prior to his arrival Elsie went out most days, taking the local bus and sometimes meeting up with friends. Recently she has been getting a bit forgetful, however, and her son has had to take on a caring role, helping her at times with personal care as well as with bills, shopping and housework. Elsie has been assessed by the care manager who has arranged for Sheila, a carer from a local agency, to call in three times a week. Sometimes Sheila finds that Elsie has left the taps on and she cannot always remember when she last ate. Once or twice there has been no food in the house and the place has been very cold. Elsie has told Sheila that on occasion she has given money to Eric but he has not returned with any groceries, spending the money at the pub. Sheila said she has seen bruises on Elsie's arms, but no explanation was forthcoming. Elsie's husband used to be physically abusive.

Following a fall at home, Elsie was admitted to hospital for a check–up, but she only had a fractured arm and it was decided that she could leave after three days. Elsie said that she was ready to go home but her daughter, who lives over 100 miles away, suggested that this would be the ideal opportunity for Elsie to move into residential accommodation nearer to her so that she could visit more regularly. Elsie is aware that her memory is not as sharp as it was, but she does not want to leave her own home. The nurses in the hospital are saying that they have to get Elsie washed and dressed as she cannot manage with her broken arm. Elsie says that with a bit of help from Sheila she could do this for herself at home. Asked about Eric, Elsie acknowledges that he can 'be a bit nasty sometimes', but that he is also a big help to her at home, and that she misses him and wants to see him when she returns home.

Case study analysis

Seeing someone like Elsie who may be vulnerable but who chooses to return to her setting can be upsetting and disturbing, and will also make practitioners aware of the level of risk and responsibility they are taking on by acquiescing with the wishes of the individual. Capacity may be an issue, but this is unlikely to be clear and uncontested. As with Elsie there may be lapses of memory, there may be risks involved in relationships, there may be genuine concerns from staff and members of the family; but think about the original question. Would a younger person be expected to go into a residential home simply because she had a broken wrist?

Policies and procedures can offer guidance on a way to manage the risk and uncertainties in a particular situation and you need to acquaint yourself with them so that you are clear about your professional responsibilities. However, as in this situation, they can provide a useful process but they will not tell you what to do. Remaining person centred in the face of uncertainty around risk, roles and capacity may involve the practitioner in taking on an advocacy role, sometimes challenging other professionals or their own or other agencies. The question of mental capacity, while often contentious, is central to the debates around best practice in the process of safeguarding vulnerable adults.

Mental capacity

It sounds as if a person-centred approach would be the best way to deal with any adult who accesses services, but there are some hard questions to consider in relation to risks and responsibilities. For example, what should practitioners do when they become aware that someone is being abused but the individual asks them not to report it? What if there is evidence of abuse but the person is too confused, scared or frail to understand or explain to anyone what has happened to them?

For adults, there is a presumption of capacity (Brown 2006). While children are assumed to have limited capacity and their well-being can and should be promoted by statutory intervention through the Children Acts 1989 and 2004 (Parton 2006), the presumption of capacity indicates that adults are autonomous individuals who have a right to make their own decisions and have ultimate authority over their own lives. In general this is not disputed. But with people who are deemed to be 'vulnerable', there is a further presumption that they may or may not be able to make their own decisions. The Mental Capacity Act (2005) tries to establish a legal framework that interferes as little as possible with an individual's rights. It highlights:

- The right of individuals to be supported to make their own decisions; this means that if someone can be given tools and information to participate in the decision-making process, these should be made available.

- The need for appropriate help to be provided before deciding that someone is unable to make their own decisions. For example, if communication is the problem rather than capacity, have the requisite interpreters or aids to communications been put in place to facilitate the person's ability to make or contribute to their own decisions?

- The right for someone to make eccentric or unwise decisions; that is, if someone makes a decision that puts them at risk but they have the capacity to make their own choices, no one should interfere with their decision. It is often the case that people will try to undermine or influence people whom they assume are vulnerable because of their age or (dis)ability (Thompson & Thompson 2005). While this may be appropriate in the case of children (although this may be disputed depending on the age and level of maturity of the young person concerned), it is not acceptable to intrude on someone else's choices in life if they have the capacity to make such choices, even where their families, friends or professionals are worried about the consequences of those choices. This, as in the case described below, can cause some difficult ethical conflicts and dilemmas for practitioners and carers.

CASE STUDY: SALLY PAYNE

Sally Payne is a 35-year-old woman with a mild to moderate learning disability and epilepsy, which is largely controlled by medication although it gets worse when she is stressed or unwell. Two years ago she moved into her own one-bedroomed flat where she lives alone, attending a day centre twice a week and supported by a worker from a care agency, who calls in three times a week to help Sally with her bills and housework. At the time of her move, Sally's parents were very concerned about her ability to cope. They keep in touch but recently she has refused to allow them to visit her as she says they are constantly criticising her and her life choices. They say that she only goes to see them occasionally, usually when she needs money.

In the past few weeks the care manager has received a number of calls from the agency carers expressing concern that Sally has 'taken up with' someone whom they describe as an 'undesirable character'. The man, Dermott, who is in his early 20s, has been known to social services in the past when he had a history of youth offending and spent two years as a child in local authority care. The carers think that he may be known to mental health services and that he is probably exploiting Sally by taking her money. Sally's parents are also very concerned that she will become pregnant and not be able to manage a baby. They say that when they have seen her she appears tired and shabbily dressed and that although she denies it, they believe her epilepsy is getting worse, which they attribute to stress caused by her relationship. Although the parents are adamant that Sally should be taken into residential care and the carers agree that 'something should be done' to protect her from Dermott, she herself says that there are no problems and that she is very happy with the situation where she can choose what she wears and not always be subject to the rules of her parents.

CHALLENGE

■ What do you think are the key issues in this situation?

■ What do you think about the views of the family and carers?

■ Do you think it is right that Sally should be expected to end her relationship with Dermott?

- What sorts of conflicts and dilemmas do the professionals have to deal with?

- If Sally had a more severe learning disability and was living in a care home rather than on her own, would the matter be different?

- If it was established that Sally did not have the capacity to understand the consequences of her decision to stay in her relationship with Dermott, what could, should or would the professionals be able to do?

Clearly, there is a difference between someone who can understand the consequences of the choices they have made and someone who cannot. This may be partly a level of cognitive development, but may also relate to the opportunities and chances the person has had to have experiences that have developed their ability to understand and resolve the complexities involved in personal relationships. Because someone has capacity does not mean that they are not vulnerable, nor does it mean that they may not be abused. Even if their capacity is limited, there are additional factors that anyone involved in making decisions on their behalf would need to take into account:

- Anything done for someone without capacity must be done with their best interests in mind.

- Whatever is done must be the least restrictive option available.

- Does anyone have any knowledge of what the person would most likely have wanted to do had they had the capacity to explain it? Have they expressed a preference when they had the capacity to do so?

Just because someone has 'lost' capacity or is deemed to be incapable of making their own decisions – that is, is unable to understand the consequences of a particular course of action – does not mean that they are any less valued as a person. If anything, it is the very time when person-centred values and attitudes are at their most critical.

What to do when you become aware that a vulnerable person has been abused

CHALLENGE

- Could Sally be defined as a vulnerable person?

- Could Dermott be defined as a vulnerable person?

CASE STUDY continued

As someone in receipt of community care services, Sally has a right under the NHS and Community Care Act 1990 to a further assessment of her needs. She will fit the criteria under the guidelines of the ADSS definition, which identifies as vulnerable those who are are elderly and frail, those who suffer from mental illness (including dementia), a physical, sensory or learning disability or have a long-term condition or severe physical illness.

It is therefore clear that Sally can be defined as a vulnerable adult because of her need for community care services. Her capacity may or may not be an issue, but in either case the pressure to find ways of managing the risks and concerns of others while remaining person centred in terms of accepting and appreciating her own perspective will challenge those around her. Whether Dermott can also be defined as a vulnerable adult is less clear as he is not at present receiving any services, though he may have done so in the past. Do you think this would make any difference to the decisions?

The next question to consider is whether Sally is being abused. Guidelines on safeguarding adults identify a number of categories of abuse, some of which may overlap with others. These include (one or more of) the following:

- Physical abuse.

- Sexual abuse.

- Emotional or psychological abuse.

- Financial abuse.

- Institutional abuse.

- Discrimination.

- Verbal abuse.

- Neglect.

In Sally's case it may not be easy to identify particular areas of abuse or to find undisputed evidence that abuse is taking place or any perception on her part that she has been abused. It is important to consider that other people may be exaggerating their concerns, either because they believe that they know what is best for Sally or because they are discriminating against Dermott because of his mental health and youth offending history. However, in view of the concerns expressed, it may be necessary for professionals to get together to have a strategy meeting or case conference to develop an action plan to monitor and manage the issues being highlighted.

It is important for professionals working with vulnerable adults to know about the policies and procedures that organisations should have in place to deal with issues around safeguarding adults (Revised Kent & Medway Multi Agency Adult Protection Policy, Protocols and Guidance, 2005). Once a decision has been taken to go down the route of adult protection, which will be decided in consultation with senior managers and/or senior practitioners within social services, it is important to consider some of the general principles involved in the process of identifying abuse and the issues that will need to be included when considering how to intervene in situations that involve safeguarding vulnerable adults.

How abuse comes to light

There are a number of ways in which abuse may become apparent. These include:

- Signs and symptoms.

- Disclosure by the person being abused.

- Disclosure by someone else.

- Witnessing abuse.

Signs and symptoms that have something in common with child abuse procedures may mean something different for adults. For example, bruising that could indicate abuse could with a frail older person result from a fall. Older people sometimes bruise very easily. However, if the bruising is of such a type (e.g. fingerprint bruising) or in such a place (such as back, neck or inner thighs) that it would be difficult to see how the individual could do this by knocking themselves, or if the explanation does not tally with the area or kind of bruising, abuse may be suspected.

Evidence of sexual activity in a vulnerable adult may or may not be interpreted as abuse. If the person is able to consent to the sexual activity, and if the person they are having the sexual encounter with is not in any position of professional trust in relation to that person, a sexual relationship may be appropriate. Individuals who are able to make their own decisions have a right to enjoy sexual relationships and a right to have a family life. However, the level of disability or vulnerability of the vulnerable adult will have a significant impact on how that relationship is perceived. If the person clearly does not have capacity to consent to a sexual relationship, then the Sexual Offences Act 2004 makes it clear that abuse has occurred.

Financial abuse is particularly hard to address. Often, particularly if the perpetrator is known to them, an older person may not want to prosecute or even confront the abuser. However, signs and symptoms may cause a good deal of concern to other people, professionals or carers who are in contact with the vulnerable adult. It may be that the house is cold; the person is losing weight possibly because there is not enough money for them to eat properly; bills are not being paid; or the person has stopped going out to activities they used to enjoy. With older people in particular, it is easy for professionals to assume that these changes are because of the person's age or increasing frailty. They may also not want to talk about it, because they are worried that they will get someone into trouble, that there will be repercussions or that the person will no longer come to see them. However, there are legal remedies such as power of attorney and declaratory relief (Martin 2007) that can help in such situations.

Because of the links highlighted earlier between power and vulnerability, abuse of any kind is very likely to have with it an element of emotional or psychological abuse. Verbal abuse, shouting at people or calling them hurtful or humiliating names, can wound as sharply as a physical attack. Withholding services or vital equipment (wheelchair, glasses, hearing aid and so on) or giving too much or too little medication can be particularly damaging. Using such methods to restrict someone's freedom of choice or movement may be part of a culture of abuse in a group situation such as a residential home. Institutional abuse can be particularly difficult to tackle, which is why there a case study later on that specifically looks at this issue. Poor practice, and the acceptance of poor practice in a climate that is not person centred, can contribute to an environment where abuse can flourish.

═══════════════ **CHALLENGE** ═══════════════

Can you think of any examples of poor practice that could lead to abuse? Have you had experience of or witnessed any of any of the following in a home or hospital setting?

■ Not using people's names (calling everyone 'pet' or 'darling').

■ Everyone going to the toilet at the same time (leaving toilet doors open).

■ Talking about someone as if they are not there.

■ Sharing out teeth and clothes rather than ensuring that everyone gets their own.

■ Not responding when being called.

■ Shouting at people when they need help or have an accident.

■ Not knocking on doors before entering someone's room.

■ Not giving them any choices in their lives, even over minor areas.

■ Removing people's walking frames so they cannot get about.

■ Not providing food or care that is culturally appropriate.

■ Giving people medication to make them 'easier to manage'.

How could you challenge these if you were working an environment where some of these were common practices?

I am sure you can think of other examples. Staff may be very pressed and such practices can often make it easier to manage people either as individuals or in groups. Ageism and generally lacking respect for people as individuals can contribute to an environment in which such poor practice can flourish. Discrimination on the grounds of someone's race, gender, age or disability may further disempower or disadvantage an individual who already has to depend on others for help with daily living tasks.

In addition to the detection of abuse through observation of poor practice or the existence of signs and symptoms, abuse may come to light through disclosure by the individual or by someone else, a carer or family member or another practitioner. In some cases you may be reluctant to report the concerns or the service user may ask you to keep the matter confidential. However, as a professional you have a duty to report concerns, even if they involve a colleague or carer with whom you have had a good relationship.

> Adults are regarded as citizens and the promotion of their rights, including the right to live a life free of abuse, is seen as the task of all who work with adults who access community care services.
>
> (Martin 2007: 34–5)

In deciding how to respond to this, there are certain factors that the person who has been informed of the abuse will need to consider.

- Do not delay. Sometimes when we don't know what to do or feel anxious about the possible outcome, we choose to do nothing. This paralysis can be extremely damaging.

- Do not start to investigate or ask leading questions: someone will be allocated to carry out the investigation and you can actually cause considerable problems that could jeopardise the outcome if you have been seen to be asking leading questions. It may also mean that the vulnerable person has been required unnecessarily to repeat and relive the abuse that has occurred.

- Listen carefully to what you are being told; on the other hand, if the person is speaking freely, let them tell their story without interruption;

- Demonstrate a sympathetic, concerned but not shocked approach; make it clear that the information will be taken seriously, that they did the right thing by disclosing to you and that there will be a response;

- Give information about what will happen next. If you are not sure what will happen in your agency, find out what you can and make sure that communication channels are clear, for instance do not discuss with people who do not need to know; find out who will keep the person informed.

- Make careful, clear, contemporaneous notes; it is best to make these as soon as possible after the conversation (*not* interview or investigation). Make the notes in ink and sign and date the written material; dates and times may be important and details of other people who have been involved in any way need to be recorded.

■ Distinguish between facts and opinions; don't forget that this could be used in a case conference or as evidence in court. You are entitled to have opinions and your professional analysis may be relevant, but your record should be firmly based on facts, with opinions clearly distinguished from factual information (e.g bruises are facts, how they happened can be written using the person's own words, but your theory about why they happened may be a matter of conjecture).

■ Make sure that you are clear about the policies and procedures that need to be followed. This may involve an adult protection alert followed by a strategy meeting to decide whether there is anything to investigate, an investigation (which may involve the police), a case conference to make decisions and think about how they will be implemented. This should involve all the relevant stakeholders.

■ Be aware of any issues that may arise in relation to additional needs around communication (e.g. speech or hearing problems or lack of English as a first language), and of the significance of other issues relation to anti-discriminatory practice such as racial, sexual or cultural differences. Consider how these may have affected the situation and how such matters may need to be addressed to enable the person to remain at the centre of the process.

■ See if there is anyone else who can confirm what you are being told; has anyone witnessed the abuse or been made aware of the allegations?

■ Consult as soon as possible with a senior member of staff.

The following case study, highlights a number of issues in relation to safeguarding vulnerable adults and also considers that there is not always just one way of dealing with a situation involving the abuse of vulnerable adults. The challenge is to maintain a person-centred perspective while working closely with other professionals and with families and carers to address a number of issues in a very worrying situation.

CASE STUDY: MRS GEORGIOU

A member of staff from Grey Oaks, a (fictionalised) residential care home for older people, phoned social services to report that when she went into wake up Mrs Georgiou, an 88-year-old resident who had been in the home for three years, she had noticed bruising along her legs and back. In addition, Mrs Georgiou seemed more than usually drowsy. Mrs Georgiou herself could not explain what had happened, partly because she was confused and partly because her main language is Greek. She did not seem in any particular distress, but the evidence clearly indicated that

---

CASE STUDY continued

something had happened to this resident in the night. The carer who reported the concerns was adamant there had been no bruising the previous evening when she had put Mrs Georgiou to bed. She said she took a particular interest in her because she was Greek and had no family to visit her after her husband died. She had spoken with Mrs Georgiou this morning, and she knew that she wanted to stay in the home.

The senior practitioner with responsibility for adult protection took the decision to visit immediately with a member of the contracts staff to look into the allegation. When she saw the extent of the bruising, she contacted the police who were on the scene within an hour. Although they could see bruises that indicated physical abuse – and some of the bruises could have indicated sexual abuse – Mrs Georgiou herself was too confused to offer any coherent account of what could have happened. The night staff were called in and questioned and although they said they had no knowledge of what had occurred, the manager of the home decided to suspend them.

Social services staff felt that this incident, alongside the concerns previously expressed by other care managers about the level of care in the home that could not be confirmed, warranted a case conference involving the home manager, relevant care managers and the Commission for Social Care Inspection. The police said that they had insufficient evidence against the staff member and as Mrs Georgiou could not identify anyone who had abused her, there was nothing they could do. The team leader who chaired the case conference argued that in view of the number and seriousness of the concerns, and the risks to other residents, the home should be closed down and all the residents moved to other establishments. The senior practitioner identified the risk of increased confusion and likely deaths among the residents that would result from a move and argued for working with the staff in the home for a limited period, with the aim of improving practice to provide a better environment for the residents.

CHALLENGE

■ Which of these approaches would you support?

■ How would you relate your preferred option to person-centred care and interprofessional working?

Case study analysis

The senior practitioner argued for a person-centred, interprofessional perspective that involved all the relevant stakeholders working together in partnership with staff in the home and the residents' carers and families where appropriate. This involved thinking about how to address all the elements that were presented at the case conference and to develop an effective action plan.

The action plan would:

- Enable the old people to remain in their familiar environment.

- Address the poor practice in the home by visiting, initially on a daily basis, to give advice and support to care staff so that they could provide a more interesting environment for the old people in their care. Carers in the home were interviewed individually and encouraged to explore their own concerns about the levels of practice.

- Develop new person-centred care plans by working closely with Mrs Georgiou and each of the other residents individually to look at strategies to address issues of concern (such as wandering, confusion, continence, hygiene, feeding, medication) and also to find areas of interest that would enhance and enable residents to become more engaged.

- Require community care managers to visit regularly to review care plans and ensure that they were being implemented.

- Work with staff to develop activities such as arranging outings for some of the older people and visits by local children, and support staff in setting up reminiscence groups and life-story work with individuals in their care.

- Also work with staff to develop their skills and confidence in speaking up about any areas of concern in relation to the residents.

- Involve family members and friends of the residents in monitoring the situation and supporting them in pursuing better conditions for residents.

- Engage district nurses in monitoring the medication and medical needs of the residents and develop strategies in conjunction with other professionals and care staff to address these so there was no need to overmedicate.

- Work with the manager and home owners to identify working practices to ensure that staff members were not left to cope without support. The home owners expressed concern about the level of practice and appointed a new manager. Although there was no formal evidence against any member of staff, the new manager changed their working patterns so that no one would be left alone with a resident. They also set up a training programme in adult protection awareness for all members of staff.

- Set up a series of unannounced visits by the Commission for Social Care Inspection for six months to monitor the action plan and report back to regular review meetings.

Conclusion

As you can see from the above, safeguarding adults can be a challenging and complex, though rewarding, area of work. Legal, ethical and professional frameworks are all likely to be involved and every case will be different from every other. The last example, which encompasses a number of issues that have arisen over the years that adult protection has been an issue in relation to older people in residential care, demonstrates how the critical issues in achieving effective outcomes with vulnerable adults will be person-centred care and interprofessional practice.

> Successful sharing of knowledge and information between professions and agencies requires the ability to communicate complex knowledge in simple ways. The avoidance of jargon and discipline specific language can aid understanding. Sharing of knowledge can lead to joint problem solving, challenging assumptions and ideologies, and result in innovative outcomes.
>
> (Barrett et al. 2005: 45)

It is clear that a student or relatively inexperienced practitioner would not be expected to take decisions individually. In determining the best course of action a number of factors have to be considered. Some of the following issues are taken from the experience of working with children (Corby 2006), although these have been reconsidered in the light of the differences involved in working with adults and the importance of person-centred care.

The issues to consider include:

- The intent of the perpetrator and the relationship between the perpetrator and the vulnerable individual. Clearly, there is a good deal of difference between the perception that someone has deliberately targeted a vulnerable adult to exploit or abuse them, rather than a situation of a carer who has reached the end of their tether coping with the emotional demands of caring for an individual who may be distressed or demanding. In one case it may be appropriate to involve the police and if necessary even remove the vulnerable person; in the other a process of counselling, respite and support may be in order.

- The seriousness of the injury, the risk of further injury and the risk to other vulnerable adults. Assessment of levels of risk and how these can be managed or addressed needs to be part of the process of determining the urgency and level of intervention. In some cases a formal risk-assessment process may be required involving one or more individuals.

- Options for intervention, the consequences of intervention and the consequences of non-intervention. Legal and procedural frameworks will inform the decision-making process. Sometimes it is not possible to predict with accuracy what will happen in a particular scenario (Phillips *et al.* 2006). At times the adult protection procedures can provide a valuable framework for monitoring and managing uncertainty.

- Person-centred care has to take into account wherever possible the wishes, choices and capacity of the individual. Although the process of safeguarding individuals is likely to be distressing and difficult, the professionals involved should always look to see if there are ways in which the experience can be used to empower and enable those at the heart of the process (Thompson 2007). Thinking about the case studies considered in this chapter, it would be possible to identify ways in which, for example, Elsie or Sally could be helped to be more proactive in clarifying what they want for themselves and how to achieve their goals. In the case of the residential home, while it is clearly most undesirable for the event to have led to the abuse of Mrs Georgiou, there were many good outcomes as a result of the abuse coming to light. Particularly where residents are vulnerable and confused, the care staff members need training to raise awareness of the possibility of abuse and be encouraged to report it when it occurs.

- Professional responsibility for all of the practitioners may involve a challenge between the duty of care required by their professional bodies and their personal commitment to the needs of people in their care and the wishes and autonomy of the individual. Legal and procedural frameworks are essential for good management of difficult situations involving the safeguarding of vulnerable adults. Fear of professional or public exposure may lead to a tendency to 'play safe' or engage in blaming each other. However, at the heart of all the issues that have to be considered in safeguarding work will be the values and attitudes of diverse practitioners, and the values and attitudes of others stakeholders (Banks 2006). Key findings from investigations into abuse and from the case studies discussed in this chapter highlight the importance of careful and respectful working among professionals from different disciplines and the necessity for engagement with other stakeholders to share risks and responsibilities.

- A social model of vulnerability and an awareness of the need to consider issues of empowerment, and ensuring that service users (and carers where appropriate) are fully informed and as involved as much as they can be in the safeguarding process, can help to transform a difficult and worrying situation into one where change, learning and development can occur. Cultural and other differences must be addressed to ensure that the person or people at the centre of any investigation are as fully involved as it is possible for them to be. In circumstances that often provoke strong emotional reactions, and that moreover make such demands on the practitioners and other people involved, it is more crucial than ever to place at the centre of the plethora of complications and considerations the rights, views and needs of the vulnerable people who may be at risk

References

Adams, R., Dominelli, L. & Payne, M. (2002) *Social Work: Themes, Issues and Critical Debates*, 2nd edn. Basingstoke: Palgrave.

Association of Directors of Social Services (2005) *Safeguarding Adults: A National Framework of Standards for Good Practice and Outcomes in Adult Protection Work*. London: Association of Directors of Social Services.

Banks, S. (2006) *Ethics and Values in Social Work*, 3rd edn. Basingstoke: Palgrave Macmillan.

Barrett, G., Sellman, D. & Thomas, J. (2005) *Interprofessional Working in Health & Social Care: Professional Perspective*. Basingstoke: Palgrave Macmillan.

Brammer, A. (2007) *Social Work Law*, 2nd edn. Harlow: Pearson Educational.

Brown, K. (ed.) (2006) *Vulnerable Adults and Community Care*. Exeter: Learning Matters.

Corby, B. (2006) *Child Abuse: Towards a Knowledge Base*, 3rd edn. Maidenhead: Open University Press.

Crawford, K. & Walker, J. (2003) *Social Work with Older People*. Exeter: Learning Matters.

Department of Health (2000) *No Secrets: Guidance on Developing and Implementing Multi Agency Policies and Procedures to Protect Vulnerable Adults from Abuse*. London: HMSO.

Johns, R. (2005) *Using the Law in Social Work*, 2nd edn. Exeter: Learning Matters.

Jowitt, M. & McLoughlin, S. (eds.) (2005) *Social Work with Children and Families*. Exeter: Learning Matters.

Kelmshall, H. & Pritchard, J. (1997) *Good Practice in Risk Assessment and Risk Management*. London: Jessica Kingsley.

Kent & Medway Revised Multi Agency Adult Protection Policy, Protocols and Guidance (2005).

Mandelstam, M. (1999) *Community Care Practice and the Law*, 2nd edn. London: Jessica Kingsley.

Martin, J. (2007) *Safeguarding Adults*. Lyme Regis: Russell House.

Oliver, M. & Sapey, B. (2006) *Social Work with Disabled People*, 3rd edn. Basingstoke: Palgrave Macmillan.

Parton, N. (2006) *Safeguarding Childhood*. Basingstoke: Palgrave Macmillan.

Philips, J., Ray, M. & Marshall, M. (2006) *Social Work with Older People*, 4th edn. Basingstoke: Palgrave Macmillan.

Swain et al. (2005) *Controversial Issues in a Disabling Society*. Maidenhead: Open University Press.

Thompson, N. (2007) *Power and Empowerment*. Lyme Regis: Russell House.

Thompson, S. & Thompson, N. (2005) *Community Care*. Lyme Regis: Russell House.

Warren, J. (2007) *Service User and Carer Participation in Social Work*. Exeter: Learning Matters.

Care for the Carers: Who is in the Centre?

Hilary Bungay and Patricia Walker

This chapter aims to:

- Define formal and informal care.

- Explore the input of formal and informal carers to person-centred care.

- Consider the support mechanisms in place for formal and informal carers in the context of institutional and community provision.

- Reflect on the importance of collaboration between formal and informal care providers.

- Consider the potential conflicts that may arise between formal state and informal care provision, and the conflicts that may exist between the cared-for person and the carer.

Caring

Care is an integral part of life. We all experience it at some time in our lives, either as the recipient of care or the giver of care, the balance changes throughout our lifespan and it is a fundamental part of being human. Care is the provision of what is necessary for health, welfare, maintenance and protection of someone. It can also mean the protective custody or guardianship by a local authority of children whose parents are either dead or unable to look after them. We talk about 'taking care' in term of being careful, or paying close attention to something so as to avoid damage or risk. We may 'care about' somebody – that is, we feel concern and feel affection for them – and when we talk about 'care for someone' we look after them and try to ensure that their needs are met and that they are safe. To feel cared for is something that most people crave: to feel loved, cherished and secure, to have someone pay attention to us and be interested in what we are doing. According to Herring (2007) caring is enriching because it forms relationships within families and the wider community and without it society would collapse.

In terms of health and social services, it is the degree of dependency that creates a need for care. A common characteristic of those needing care is that their condition is not curable, be it chronic illness, disability, age-related frailty, learning disabilities or mental health problems. As a consequence, there is a potential cost of long-term use of medical and social services; needs are often multiple and are not the responsibility of a single profession or agency (Allsop 1995). Effective interagency and interprofessional working is required to promote planned care that addresses the many dimensions of the individual's care needs. Professional practitioners need to communicate effectively with each other, and understand each other's roles to be able to adapt to changing care needs. This has to include active collaboration with the patient/client and their family and/or friends.

Twigg and Atkin (1994) conceptualised caring in terms of a combination of elements. For them care involves:

- The performance of tasks beyond those normally expected; that is, doing things for people that they cannot do for themselves, often involving hard physical labour.

- Caring almost always takes place within a context of kinship that is within the family.

- Carers do not simply do the physical tasks but they also support those for whom they care emotionally.

- Caring involves a feeling of being responsible for the cared-for person. This sense of responsibility is rooted within the obligations of the relationship and carers are bound into the relationship, which means that they do not simply give up when the balance of interest turns against continuing.

Throughout this book the focus has been on person-centred care. The person-centred approach recognises and seeks to address the multiple and inseparable influences that affect an individual's health. People who 'care' seek to understand an individual's needs by involving them and integrating their input to care planning, which may involve a range of formal professional and informal input.

Formal and informal carers: A definition

For the purpose of this chapter, carers have been identified to be of two main types, formal and informal. A formal carer includes any person who receives payment due to being employed or self-employed in the provision of health or social care services, for example social workers, midwives, nurses, radiographers, care assistants, therapists and doctors. An informal carer is someone who provides physical or social support for a relative or friend and in their absence or in the absence of other informal carer support, intervention from health, social or the voluntary sector would be required (May *et al.* 2001); informal carers are unpaid.

The name 'carer' has been generally accepted by politicians, service providers and indeed the general public, yet for some scholars it has powerful connotations because it identifies and labels activities that until the 1970s and 1980s were invisible and taken for granted as a part of family life (Parker & Clarke 2002). Traditionally the literature identifies an informal carer as a person who has been identified as a key carer, possibly after a 'carer's assessment'. However, although this distinction exists, the term 'informal carer' is actively disliked by many carers (Clements 2007), because they feel that there is actually nothing informal about the level of care they provide or indeed the amount of time they devote to it. Referring to caring as involuntary or informal also makes it seems less important.

Similarly, consider the term 'cared-for person' within the 'caring' relationship when one person is dependent on another. How does it feel in this position to be the 'cared-for' person or labelled as dependent? There is a tension between carers and the disability movement and their respective influences over policy. Parker and Clarke (2002) maintain that disabled and older people may see 'carer' as a derogatory term, as it suggests dependence and immaturity; furthermore, it suggests that the person requires care at all times, whereas in reality the level of help required is variable with time and circumstances.

In deference to those expressed feelings, throughout this chapter unpaid carers will be referred to as 'carers' rather than informal carers, and all paid carers will be referred to as health and social care practitioners. Some may prefer to be called health or social care professionals, but there are many paid carers who are employed through direct payments who may not have any qualifications and so from some perspectives would not be classed as professionals; there are people in the voluntary sector who fulfil caring roles that are neither paid nor fit within the traditional view of a carer. However, this chapter is not the place to debate what constitutes a professional or theories of professionalisation and for simplicity's sake, while recognising and respecting these views, the terms 'carers' and 'health and social care practitioners' are adopted. You may like to consider alternative terms for 'cared-for person', 'carer' and 'practitioners'. Are there terms or names that would be preferable that describe the situation and relationship between those involved?

Who are the carers?

Carers look after family; partners or friends in need of help because they are ill, frail or have a disability. The care they provide is unpaid.

(Carers UK 2001)

Gender differences exist in attitudes to caring: women tend to view caring as a normal part of their lives (Gattuso & Bevan 2000), while men may perceive caring to be an additional role (Fisher 1994). Demographically, most informal carers are female, aged over 60, caring for a spouse or adult child. An analysis of census records found that most carers are middle-aged woman who have multiple roles within the family (Dahlberg *et al.* 2007). Many of these women are providing care for a sick or disabled child and are 'heavy end' carers; that is, they provide more than 50 hours of care a week in a long-term care situation (Yeandle *et al.* 2007a). However, many carers are elderly males aged 80–89 in a spousal relationship with the person receiving care, yet they themselves are often frail (Dahlberg *et al.* 2007). Few studies have explored informal care provision among minority ethnic groups in the UK, but a small survey of African/Caribbean carers identified an acceptance of caring as part of life's biography. The pre-caring role was viewed as continuous with that of caring, albeit highly disruptive to relationships within the family (Adamson & Donovan 2005).

There are also people under the age of 18 who undertake a caring role, 'young carers' (Department of Health 1999). They provide care for their mother/stepmother, father/stepfather, sibling, grandparent or other person who has a range of conditions including physical disabilities, mental health problems and learning disabilities, and sensory impairment. Young carers undertake a range of caring tasks including domestic work (cooking, cleaning and washing), general nursing care such as giving medication, changing dressings and assisting with mobility. Some undertake intimate tasks involving personal care, while other care is supportive of mental health needs. Other activities undertaken by young carers include translating for non-English-speaking relatives, accompanying on hospital visits, paying household bills and other administrative roles. Few projects have explored the time allocated by young carers to their caring role, however Dearden and Becker (2004a) identified a range of less than 5 hours to over 50 hours spent caring per week. It is important to recognise, therefore, that carers are not a homogeneous group, and that carers can be men, women and children from all social and ethnic groups; as such they will have diverse needs.

The impact of caring

The adoption of a caring role can result in significant lifestyle changes and can create difficulties for the carer. Carers face a number of disadvantages. They suffer financially if they give up work or reduce their working hours to undertake care; this also has implications for their future pension and may result in them living in poverty as an older person. There is a close relationship between the health of the carer and hours of care given (Power *et al.* 2007); carers who are particularly vulnerable to poor health are those providing care in excess of 35 hours per week (Yeandle *et al.* 2007a). Yeandle *et al.* (*ibid.*) found that carers who are in poor health themselves, have no formal qualifications, are providing care in excess of 20 hours per week and are caring for a child under

19 years or for a person with a learning disability or mental health problem experience even greater financial difficulties. The health of a carer can be affected physically as a result of having to lift the cared-for person, not being able to get exercise and a poor diet due to time constraints and relative poverty. They may also suffer from anxiety and depression due to the responsibility of giving another person full-time care, and being isolated and excluded from the community. Young carers have been found to disadvantaged educationally and socially. High levels of caring may reduce social activities for young carers, including time with friends and for leisure. The transition to adulthood may be more difficult, as there has been less time for school and home work. Many young carers miss school time and experience educational difficulties, especially in the 11–15 age group (Dearden & Becker 2004a, 2004b).

Carers may also face a challenge to their personal identity. Having defined themselves through life in roles such as a wife, husband, daughter, son or other related person or partner, or through their employment, religion or hobbies, now their life situation has changed. While they may be able to retain some of these roles, becoming a carer creates another and different label with which they may or may not be comfortable. Indeed, Tomkinson (2006) comments, 'in official jargon, at case conferences and on social services forms, I become a carer and he [my husband], becomes my cared for. As if we hadn't always cared for, or about each other.' Carers do want to be seen as individuals in their own right. As a respondent to a questionnaire researching carers' experiences of hospital support stated, they want 'to be treated like a person and not just as carer' (Bungay & Alaszewski 2003).

Being a carer is not always without its benefits. The cared-for person may provide love, gratitude and emotional support for the carer (Fine & Glendinning 2005 in Herring 2007). Indeed, carers and the cared-for person may well support each other in mutual caring roles, whereby the ymonitor each other's physical and mental well-being, which in turn influences their personal interactions (Henderson & Forbat 2002). Care has a strong emotional component; for the person providing care this can be 'emotional labour', which has been likened to physical labour in the sense that it is labour as in hard work (James 1992). This occurs at times when a gap exists between what was felt and what the person hoped to feel. Emotional labour has been explained as the management and regulation of feeling (Hochschild 1983), involving:

> the suppression of feeling in order to sustain the outward appearance that produces the proper state of mind in others – that of being cared for in a safe and convivial place.
>
> (Hochschild 1983: 7)

According to James (1992), the 'labourer' is expected to respond to another person and the response is shaped by the care interactions between the carer and cared-for person. Hochschild (1983) identified several criteria that enable emotional engagement to take place in a care interaction, including face-to-face or voice contact with another person and an ability to produce an emotional state, for example gratitude in that person. The quality of the care interactions within the relationship has a significant impact on the physical and psychological stress experienced, with those who have had a poor relationship perceiving their caring role as burdensome and interpreting the situation in a negative way (Thompson *et al.* 1990). For example, a carer described her bitterness, anger and despair providing care for a 98-year-old mother:

> Why do I find it impossible to nurse this needy, wreckage of a human being, who has taken over my life, with a genuinely selfless good heart. A relationship that may have been loving has become one of hate – Everything about her revolts me now.
>
> (Family Secrets 2007)

This demonstrates how caring relations can potentially be very fragile: even the most devoted can break down due to demands on time, loss of energy and drained personal resources. Yet the woman who wrote this piece refused to place her mother in a care home through concern that she would not be properly cared for.

While many carers are devoted to the person for whom they care, the caring role can also be adopted because there is a sense of obligation and guilt. A sense of obligation may lead to a repeated commitment to care in difficult circumstances and people may try to overcome the guilt they feel at their resentment by renewed caring – 'it is the guilt of this that binds me to this living hell' (Family Secrets 2007). Guilt has been identified as one of the most personal human emotions, which can tear individuals apart emotionally (Gaylin 1985). It can be a particular dilemma for spousal carers, especially when it comes to accepting respite care and the feeling that they are disloyal for sending their partner away (Arksey & Glenndinning 2006).

CASE STUDY: JOHN AND EILEEN

John and Eileen Venner are a couple in their early 80s who have been identified by their GP as having problems at home. He thinks that Mrs Venner has some short-term memory loss and as Mr Venner is not able to cope with her, she may need to be placed in a residential home.

When visited by a social worker, Mr Venner is vocal in his complaints that his wife is no longer able to manage the cooking and housework and says he has to do everything for her. Mrs Venner is generally quiet, but whenever she does try to speak Mr Venner interrupts her and tells the social worker to ignore her, as she doesn't know what she is saying. When the possibility of residential care is mentioned, Mr Venner insists that he doesn't want his wife to go away and Mrs Venner starts to cry.

■ What issues does this scenario raise for you?

■ How do you perceive the relationship between Mr and Mrs Venner?

■ Who needs more help, Mr or Mrs Venner?

■ What help could be given as an alternative to residential care for Mrs Venner?

■ Consider this scenario in relation to the Adult Protection issues raised in Chapter 7.

Case study analysis

In this case Mr Venner states that he wants his wife to remain at home, in which case services could be provided at home to help relieve his situation. This could be at the expense of Mrs Venner, the cared-for person. Would she be happier (and safer?) if she was in a residential home? It also raises uncertainty about who is in the centre when we talk about person-centred care. If the focus is on the cared-for person the carer's needs may be neglected and, conversely, if the carer's needs are the focus the cared-for person's needs may not be met. Therefore person-centred care requires an approach in which the interests of both the carer and the cared for are considered together. The interests of the carer and the cared for should be seen as interlinking rather than competing.

Within the caring role a number of potential conflicts may arise between the carer, the cared-for person and practitioners: lack of information regarding services; lack of training; issues of confidentiality; feelings of isolation and abandonment; financial problems; sense of responsibility and anxiety; lack of communication between different agencies.

■ Why do you think these may be sources of conflict?

■ Can you think of other sources of potential conflict?

Consider these potential conflicts and, as you proceed, try to think whether the policies and strategies the government has introduced to support carers could resolve some or all of them.

The evolution of care systems and the impact on person-centred care

At the beginning of the nineteenth century in the UK there was minimal health or welfare provision by the state. There were voluntary and charitable hospitals and workhouses that provided some level of health and social care, and the wealthy had private physicians for their medical care. The middle and upper classes did not tend to go into the hospitals and provision for the working classes was very much dependent on where in the country they lived (the postcode lottery of care has always existed). Caring for the sick was therefore generally carried out by family members. It was not until the 1911 National Insurance Health Act that the state became involved in providing personal health services, and with the inception of the NHS in 1948 health care became increasing institutionalised, with care being provided in hospitals. Scientific medicine and the medical profession were dominant, and the evolving technology in medicine led to the tendency for patients to be perceived in terms of their condition or illness rather than holistically. Towards the end of the twentieth century there was a move to empower patients and recognise their right to autonomy, but to achieve this in the context of the law meant creating an image of isolated individual patients (Herring 2007). Consequently, we have seen a paradigm shift in health care from person to patient to person, but the residual perception of a stand-alone patient coupled with the prevailing view of caring as women's work means that it was not given recognition or respect. As a result of this, carers and their contributions were invisible to the government and policy makers.

Since the 1960s, successive governments have emphasised the need to provide community care. The main objective is to enable individuals to remain in their own homes, rather than being cared for in long-stay institutions or residential establishments. The initial emphasis was on 'care in' the community, but during the 1970s there was a shift to 'care by' the community (Finch 1990 cited in Allen 2000). By the end of the 1970s informal family care was the mainstay of community care. This was the result of a number of financial, social and political influences: the ageing population, public expenditure contraction, the Left-wing perspective that institutional care was repressive, and Right-wing policies on individual responsibility and family values (Allen 2000). The implementation of government policies has gradually shifted the balance of responsibility for meeting users' ongoing care needs from the hospitals and institutions to the community. The emphasis has been on enabling people with continuing care needs to be discharged home from hospital wherever possible, without unnecessary delays and discontinuities in their care (Heaton *et al.* 1999).

Despite the dependence on and expectations of community carers, carers were not mentioned in social care legislation until the 1986 Disabled Persons (Services, Consultation and Representation) Act, although since then their recognition by government has risen dramatically (Clements 2007). Britain has an estimated six million carers and one in six households (17 per cent) contains a carer (Department of Health 2005). The economic value of the contribution made by carers in the UK is £87 billion per year (Buckner & Yeandle 2007), which is more than the annual costs of all aspects of the NHS, audited in 2006–07 as £81.67 billion (Department of Health 2007).

'Carers as a resource' (Twigg & Atkin 1994) has been the predominate care model on which government policy has been based. Twigg and Atkin identify four models of response that service providers adopt towards carers:

■ *Carers as resources.* In this model there is an assumption among service providers that in some sense informal care comes first, and that there is only a need for the social care system to step in when informal care is unavailable. This model places the cared-for person at the centre of focus and the carer only features as part of the background.

■ *Carers as co-workers.* In contrast to the carers as resources model, this sees the carers' interests and well-being being considered by the providers. However, this is essentially on an instrumental basis and the primary aim is to provide high-quality care for the cared-for person.

■ *Carers as co-clients.* Under this model, carers are regarded as people in need of help in their own right and services are provided with the aim of relieving their situation and enhancing their morale. Support is aimed at those who are most highly stressed and in some cases the interests of the carer are pursued at the expense of the cared-for person.

■ *Superseded carers.* The final model sees the carer being replaced in the caregiving relationship. This may be due to concern for the independence of the cared-for person or out of concern for the carer. In these cases the term 'carer' is replaced by 'family' or 'relatives', which are less evocative of the level of responsibility assigned to the role of the carer.

These models, however, do not really fit within the concept of person-centred care, as in three the carer's needs are viewed as separate from the cared-for person. To assess the carer as a 'co-client' suggests or labels the carer as someone who is need of help, yet if they were not undertaking the caring role it is possible that they would not be seen as clients or even have contact with the service provider. An alternative model of response that service providers could adopt towards the carer would be a collaborative or partnership model; that is, one that sees the service user and carer as participants in the process of supporting and enabling both, a collaboration that involves both users and cares in decisions about the services they receive. In effective person-centred care, carers who want and are able to continue their role should have their needs considered in conjunction with the cared-for person.

The situation and circumstances of carers can vary depending on the nature of the onset of care and the duration for which they have been providing it (Yeandle *et al.* 2007b). New carers experience significant changes to their lives. Sometimes care support may develop gradually as the health of a family member, relative or friend progressively deteriorates. This pattern of care development enables the carer to identify sources of help and advice and to adjust to changing circumstances. For others, caring responsibilities occur suddenly as a result of an accident, stroke or unanticipated health alteration.

CASE STUDY: MR AND MRS BROWN

Mr Brown has been acutely ill in hospital requiring intensive care. He is now on a medical ward and has a tracheotomy *in situ*, but has been pronounced fit for discharge and is desperate to return home. His wife has been shown how to use suction to clear the tracheotomy and is willing for Mr Brown to return home, but only on the understanding that the district nursing team will visit every day to assess him and monitor his airway.

On Friday afternoon Mr Brown returns home and over the weekend Mrs Brown is expecting visits from the GP and the nursing team. However, no one arrives and she is unable to make contact with anyone in the local GP Practice. She phones the hospital and receives reassurance from the staff; although she remains very anxious she manages to cope, and Mr Brown's condition appears to remain stable. First thing on Monday morning she phones the GP Practice, who say they were unaware that Mr Brown had been discharged and that they were expected to visit. There had evidently been some communication breakdown.

CHALLENGE

■ How could this situation have been avoided?

■ Where could Mrs Brown have accessed help or support?

■ What level of nursing care would you anticipate a carer to be able to manage at home?

■ What are the potential consequences for Mrs Brown and her willingness to care for her husband in the future?

Government policies and strategies introduced to support carers

During the 1980s there were a number of reviews of community care that identified an overall lack of strategy. For example, the Audit Commission (1986) and the Griffiths Report (1988) found that arrangements for community care were in disarray. In response to these criticisms, the government published *Caring for People* (Department of Health and Social Security 1989). This put particular stress on supporting care givers in practical ways to enable people to stay at home, and was therefore a major shift in health and social care policy. It moved carers from a position in the wings where they were virtually ignored to one where they were almost centre stage (Baldwin & Parker 1989 cited in Pickard 2001).

The proposals in *Caring for People* were implemented in the 1990 NHS and Community Care Act. The Act required local authorities to take account of carers when undertaking assessments of needs. The key objective for service delivery was that 'service providers make practical support for carers a high priority'. However, this concern for carers was essentially instrumental, with the knowledge that helping carers to maintain their contribution to care was a sound investment (Pickard 2001). Family carers therefore continued to be seen as a resource and the measures were primarily aimed to 'keep carers caring'.

The government responded to further political lobbying with The Carers (Recognition and Services) Act (1995), which for the first time provided certain carers with a statutory right to an assessment of need (Nolan 2001). However, the Act was limited in a number of ways: no rights to services were conferred on carers and they could not request an assessment unless the person for whom they were caring was also being assessed. In addition, to be eligible for assessment carers had to be providing substantial care on a regular basis, however neither 'substantial' nor 'regular' was defined and so could be subject to interpretation. Furthermore, no additional resources accompanied the Act, so local authorities struggled to address carers' needs in the face of competing demands (Nolan 2001). Evaluation of the Carers (Recognition and Services) Act found its implementation to be piecemeal and patchy (Nolan 2001) and realisation that the Act was only partially effective resulted in the launch of the Carers National Strategy, *Caring about Carers* (Department of Health 1999). This was intended to mark a substantial shift in policy and culture so that carers were not only recognised but also respected and admired. The primary objective of the strategy was:

> focussed on enabling those who choose to care, and those whose care is wanted by another person, to do so without detriment to the carer's inclusion in society and to their health. Our aim is to support people who choose to be carers.
>
> (Department of Health 1999)

The Carers (Recognition and Services) Act thus failed to address the well-being of carers in their own right. This was addressed later in the Carers and Disabled Children Act (2000), which extended the rights of carers, giving them the right to an assessment of their needs even where the cared-for person has refused an assessment for, or the provision of, community care services, provided the cared-for person would be eligible for community care services. Neither the 1995 nor the 2000 Act placed any direct obligation on the NHS to support the needs of carers (Clements 2007). However, the Practice Guidance to the 1995 Act did advise that staff working in primary care were well placed to notice carer stress and therefore should be aware of the services available to carers and should inform the carer of their rights. Likewise, it was suggested that social services departments should ensure that primary care staff have the relevant information regarding social services criteria and how to make a referral.

In 1999 the Royal Commission on Long Term Care reported and recommended that government should 'ensure that services become increasingly "carer blind"', meaning that 'the existence of a carer will not lead to the failure to offer services' as a means of providing support to the carer. The National

Strategy for Carers, in contrast, emphasised the development of systems to provide carers with short breaks. Yet such short breaks or respite can also be a source of conflict for carers: they may recognise they need a break but are unhappy with the quality of available care, or are concerned about the impact on the cared-for person, including deterioration in their condition. They may also be worried that it signals to family and community that they are unable to cope (Ashworth & Baker 2000).

The third major policy relating to carers was the Carers (Equal Opportunities) Act (2004). This marked a cultural shift in the ways in which carers were perceived, from unpaid providers of care services to people in their own right, with the right to work and to take part in education and leisure activities. This placed an obligation on social services to inform carers of their rights and to require carers' assessments to consider whether the carer works or wishes to work, and/or is undertaking or wishing to undertake education, training or leisure activities. However, this is still essentially aimed at supporting carers within their caring role rather than replacing them with paid carers.

Further consideration of carers appeared in *Your Health, Your Care, Your Say* (Department of Health 2005), with the government promising to update the Carers' Strategy to reflect developments in carers' rights, direct payments, carers' assessments and grants. *Your Health, Your Care, Your Say* included a 'New Deal for Carers' to develop a cross-government strategy that promotes the health and well-being of carers in recognition that people who are caring for more than 50 hours per week are twice as likely not to be in good health as those who are not carers, that three-quarters of carers are worse off financially because of their caring responsibilities, and that 400 000 carers combine full-time work with caring for more than 20 hours per week. The 'New Deal' encourages councils and primary care trusts to nominate a lead for carers' services, pledges to establish an information/helpline for carers, to ensure that short-term home-based respite support is supplied for carers in a crisis or emergency situation in all council areas, and to allocate funding for the creation of an expert carers' programme to provided training for carers to develop skills. The introduction of an information line is potentially very important, because of the six million carers in the UK at any one time it is generally not appreciated that this is a rapidly changing group, with approximately two million adults becoming (and ceasing to be) carers every year (Hirst 2001 in Clements 2007). This evidently has major implications for informing people of available services and their rights.

Policies and guidance for supporting carers have also been produced for social services. The New Outcomes Framework for Performance Assessment of Adult Social Care (Commission for Social Care Inspection 2006) aimed to place carers at the centre of adult care services, making carers a core client group alongside older people, people with learning disabilities, mental health and physical and sensory disability (Clements 2007). In addition to passing legislation in the form of Acts, the government has produced practice guidance to assist in their implementation (Department of Health 1995, 2000, 2004; SCIE 2004).

The practice guidance (Department of Health 1995, 2000) also considers the concept of autonomy in the context of the caring relationship. First, the assumption should not be made that the carer is willing to continue caring; secondly, assumptions should not be made about the nature of tasks that a carer is willing to undertake, particularly those related to personal intimate care. Although it is important to consider this from the carer's perspective, it also paramount to consider it from the cared-for person's perspective too. The cared-for person may not wish to have personal activities such as bathing and dressing performed by a close family member, feeling that it is intrusive and inappropriate; they may prefer to have a more detached form of help (Brechin 2000).

CASE STUDY: MAURICE LONG AND MRS MEADOWS

Maurice Long, aged 30, has requested help with regard to the care option for his mother, Mrs Meadows, aged 45. Mrs Meadows has had multiple sclerosis for 17 years and needs a lot of assistance with her everyday personal care. Since his father left some years ago Maurice has been performing much of this care, but now feels that the situation has become too emotionally and physically demanding for him and is unable to cope.

Mrs Meadows, on the other hand, will not accept outside 'interference' in her personal care and she says that Maurice is the only person who understands her needs. She feels that Maurice is being selfish and wants to leave her because she has given him all her money in return for looking after her and she is now in debt. Mrs Meadows is very distressed and says that if her son abandons her she will have nothing left to live for.

CHALLENGE

- Consider the care dynamics in this relationship.

- What are the family issues?

- Who rights should be prioritised in this situation?

- Who decided what the problem is?

- How could this situation be resolved?

- How do recent policy changes potentially benefit Maurice?

We can see, therefore, that the government has introduced a number of policies and strategies to support carers. Yet most government policies fail to recognise the multidimensional nature of care, and in particular the polarisation of the needs of the patient and carer (Lloyd 2000). From the perspective of policy, care is the defining element, whereas the carer views their interpersonal relationship with the patient as central (Henderson & Forbat 2002). Recent policy has in theory given equal consideration of carers' individual requirements alongside those of the patients. However, the plethora of policy and legislation does not necessarily mean that carers get the support they require or need.

Research has found that a priority for carers is for health and social services to work together to provide a seamless service (Henwood 1998). The Combined Policy Guidance (Department of Health 2005a) recommends that social services and their NHS partners should develop a multi-agency carers' strategy to help support carers. This is where effective interprofessional collaboration is key: professionals from all services need to have an inherent understanding of each other's roles and responsibilities to be able to deliver the necessary support for carers.

The level of health and social services support to carers is varied and not all interventions are of use. While most studies suggest only a temporary improvement in carer health following increased support (Forster & Young 1996; Geddes & Chamberlain 1994), some interventions have proved beneficial. Valuable interventions include the provision of occupational therapy (Logan et al. 1997) and a family social worker (Dennis et al. 1997). However, Edmonds (2007: 8) identified the requirement to 'fight for everything' in a struggle to meet needs. Particular problems included poorly coordinated, discontinuous care with little information about available services, aids, adaptations, welfare benefits and 'end-of-life' planning. Yet without the input of carers, many sick, disabled or older people would be unable to cope.

Power relationships in care provision

Within any relationship there is the potential for an imbalance of power to exist. According to Laverack (2005), power suffuses relationships between professional practitioners and their patients, and can be used in such relationships 'with others' or 'over others'. Power over others can be positive or negative. Positive power involves effective use of knowledge, skills, expertise, information and resources to improve care provision; conversely, negative power may seek to limit or restrict the care provided, possibly using coercion. Practitioners hold a specialised body of knowledge and this gives them power, which can be used positively to the greater good of the care recipient, but there is also the potential for the practitioner to use this knowledge to create a distance between them as expert and the client (Turner 1987). This distance can exist between the practitioner and the cared-for person but also between the practitioner and the carer. Just as there are expert patients or clients who are experts in managing their own condition (Department of Health 2001b), so there are carers who have a special knowledge of the cared-for person's needs. This knowledge is a result of caring for the person over a long period, sharing experiences with other carers and, for some, using the internet to expand their knowledge of the cared-for person's condition. Carers do often see themselves as experts and therefore as advocates for the cared-for person; if they do not feel that they are listened to, this can engender a feeling of powerlessness and helplessness. Some practitioners may find 'expert' carers threatening and this can result in conflict, especially if the carer does not feel that they are listened to, as this carer of a young disabled adult expressed about an incident that had arisen on a hospital ward:

> I feel sorry for the medical profession because they have to be on their guard all the time but they could gain enormous rewards when you think we have been caring for that person for years, 24 hours a day, we are willing to come in we are not there to criticise we are in fact there to co-operate.
>
> (Bungay & Alaszewski 2003)

Carers do want to be involved in the decision-making process concerning the treatment or resource allocation to the cared-for person, not only because they are concerned for the welfare of that person but also because decisions will have an impact on their lives as well. This falls within the 'ethic of care' referred to in Chapter 3 in regard to respect for autonomy. The ethic of care perspective (Tronto 1993) would take into account the carer's position in the cared-for person's life narrative and, rather than promoting independent decision making, would encourage decisions to be made through communication with all those involved in the caring relationship. However, practitioners may use the issue of confidentiality, or hide behind the concept of patient or client-centred care, to preclude the carer from discussions and subsequent decision making. This could be particularly difficult if it is in relation to discharge from a hospital or mental health unit, because if discharge is dependent on there being another person available to provide care at home, that person's ability to provide care and at what level needs to be established and not assumed.

Practitioners are also able to exert power as gatekeepers to resources, treatment and services. If during an assessment social services first determine what the carer is willing and able to provide in terms of care before explaining what services are available, or simply tell people that they can only have certain services, or restrict choice to a limited range of the actual services that are in theory available, then this is not only a form of implicit rationing, it is also a form of control that disempowers the carer.

There is also the potential for carers to exert power over the cared-for person. This can manifest itself in a number of ways and can constitute abuse. Abuse can be physical, such as inflicting pain, or through acts of omission, for example not cleaning the person when they are soiled. Abuse can also be emotional, bullying, exclusion from family and social life life or threatening to stop caring and place the person in a residential home (see Chapter 7 for a detailed examination of abuse and protection issues). It is not only the carer who has the ability to exercise power within the caring relationship: the cared-for person may also use feelings of guilt and obligation to ensure continued caring by the carer.

Health and social care practitioners

We have considered the support mechanisms that are in place for unpaid carers, but health and social care professionals may also require support to enable them to continue in their caring role. Approximately 1.3 million people were employed in the NHS in England in September 2005. This included 679 157 professionally qualified clinical staff (doctors, dentists, nurses, midwives, therapists and so on), 376 219 staff in support to clinical staff (nursing assistants, helpers, clerical and administrative staff) and 220 387 staff involved in the NHS infrastructure (Department of Health 2006). Therefore approximately 84 per cent of those in NHS are front-line staff with direct contact with people requiring some level of care. Social care workers represent the largest workforce in England, 4–6 per cent of the total working population, but it is a highly fragmented workforce with over 39 000 employers. It is estimated that there are approximately 1.5 million social care workers in England (Ward 2007 cited in Cole 2007). There is therefore a huge workforce of people who are employed to deliver health and social services.

All professionally qualified staff in the NHS, private health care and social services are regulated by national government policy. Everything we do in health and social care is directed by central government and, as professionals, we also are regulated by our professional organisations. Although government and professional bodies have a role in regulating our practice, they also provide a support role for workers, giving protection through legislation and policy not only for the recipients of our care but also for individual practitioners (see Table 8.1).

From Table 8.1 we can see that there are many levels of support available to practitioners in the workplace. We can contrast this to the support available to carers who care and perform tasks at home that for many are akin to those that take place on a hospital ward, for instance lifting and bathing the cared-for person. Staff on a ward are trained in lifting and manual handling techniques and are provided with assistive devices, yet a carer at home may struggle alone to change beds and dress the cared-for person. We can see that despite the numerous policies aimed at supporting carers that the government has put in place since the early 1990s, the reality is that in comparison to those in paid employment, carers do not have access to the same level of protection or support. It would be difficult for a carer to use the Health and Safety at Work legislation to improve their conditions at home or to cite European Directives over how many hours they devote each day to providing care.

Practitioners are often working as part of a team and therefore have peer support: if they are unsure about an action they can ask for help and advice. Social workers have a formal system of supervision that ensures that staff at all levels meet regularly with a supervisor to discuss cases; this also provides an opportunity to share and 'offload' emotional issues that may arise through the course of their work. Increasingly, preceptorships have been put in place where newly qualified staff in the NHS are provided with a preceptor or mentor to whom they can turn for professional advice. The NHS also provides a confidential counselling service for its staff: individuals can be referred through

Table 8.1 The range of support mechanisms existing for health and social care practioners.

Support	Level	Mechanism (examples)
Legislation	European National	Working Directives Human rights Health and Safety at Work Employment rights
Policy	National Local	NHS Plan Improving Working Lives Agenda for Change Local guidelines Standard operating procedures Occupational health
Regulatory bodies	National	Health Professions Council (HPC) Nursing and Midwifery Council (NMC) General Medical Council (GMC) General Social Care Council (GSCC)
Professional bodies Unions	National Local	British Association of Social Workers (BASW) Society of Radiographers (SOR) British Association of Occupational Therapists College of Occupational Therapists (BACOT) UNISON
Peer support	Local	Mentors Preceptorships Supervisors

the occupational health department but they can also self-refer, although use of such a service will depend on the recognition of a problem.

Carers in the community, in contrast, are often isolated and have described how sometimes family and friends disappear over time, which contributes to their isolation (Bungay & Alaszewski 2003). There is a national association, Carers UK, which has a website providing information services for carers, and there are local organisations that offer information and respite services. Support groups are also available for carers that do offer mutual support and the chance to meet people in a similar position; however, to be able to attend such a group the carer may require a respite service so that they feel comfortable leaving the cared-for person.

In conclusion, we can see from the above that the government has put in place a plethora of policies and strategies aimed at supporting carers. Nevertheless, the actual support provided to carers is in essence instrumental, in that the focus remains on helping and encouraging them to continue in their caring role. Although there is some financial recompense for carers, many long-term carers may experience financial hardship as a result of the loss of paid employment, as well as health problems due to undertaking the caring role.

======================== **CHALLENGE** ========================

■ What would happen to health and social care services if all carers were granted the same employment rights as health and social care practitioners?

■ Should there be an obligation on family members to provide care?

■ Who could provide an alternative source of care?

■ Who should pay for it?

■ If you required care in your home, which individual would you choose to care for you?

■ What characteristics does this person have that makes you think they would be best to take on this role?

References

Adamson, J. & Donovan, J. (2005) 'Normal disruption': South Asian and African/Caribbean relatives caring for an older family member in the UK. *Social Science and Medicine*, 60(1); 37–48.

Allen, D. (2000) Negotiating the role of expert carers on an adult hospital ward, *Sociology of Health and Illness*, 22(2): 149–71.

Allsop, J. (1995) *Health Policy and the NHS: Towards 2000*. 2nd edn. London: Longman.

Arksey, H. & Glendinning, C. (2006) Choice in the context of informal care-giving. *Health and Social Care in the Community*, 15(2): 165–75.

Ashworth, M. & Baker, A. H. (2000) 'Time and space': Carers' views about respite care. *Health and Social Care in the Community*, 8(1): 50–56.

Audit Commission (1986) *Making a Reality of Community Care*. London: HMSO.

Baldwin, S. & Parker, G. (1989) The Griffiths Report on community care. In M. Brenton & C. Ungerson (eds) *Social Policy Review 1988–9*, Harlow: London.

Brechin, A. (2000) The challenges of caring relationships. In A. Brechin, H. Brown & M. A. Ely (eds) *Critical Practice in Health and Social Care*. London: Open University Press/Sage.

Buckner, L. & Yeandle S. (2007) *Valuing Carers: Calculating the Value of Unpaid Care*. London: Carers UK.

Bungay, H. & Alaszewski, A. (2003) *Informal Carers: An Evaluation of Their Experiences of Hospital Support*. Study Centre for Health Service Studies University of Kent, www.kent.ac.uk/CHSS.

Carers UK (2001) *A Report on the Chances of Becoming a Carer*, Carers UK, available at www.carersuk.org

Clements, L. (2007) *Carers and Their Rights, The Law Relating to Carers*, 2nd edn. London: Carers UK.

Cole (2007) In search of the invisible workers. *The Guardian*, Wednesday 17 October.

Commission for Social Care Inspection (2006) *A New Outcomes Framework for Performance Assessment of Adult Social Care (2006–07)*. Consultation document, August. London: Commission for Social Care Inspection.

Dahlberg, L., Demack, S. & Bambra, C. (2007) Age and gender of informal carers: A population-based study in the UK. *Health and Social Care in the Community*, 15(5): 7.

Dearden, C. & Becker, S. (2004a) *Young Carers in the UK: The 2004 Report*. London: Carers UK.

Dearden, C. & Becker, S. (2004b) *Young Carers and Education*. London: Carers UK.

Dennis, M., O'Rourke, S., Slattery, J., Staniforth, T. & Warlow, C. (1997) Evaluation of stroke family care worker: Results of a randomised controlled trial. *British Medical Journal*, 314: 1071–6.

Department of Health and Social Security (1989) *Caring for People: Community Care in the Next Decade and Beyond*, Cm 849, London: HMSO.

Department of Health (1990) *The NHS and Community Care Act*, London: Department of Health.

Department of Health (1991) *Patients Charter*. London: Department of Health.

Department of Health (1995) *The Carers (Recognition and Services) Act*. London: Department of Health.

Department of Health (1999) *Caring for Carers, Carers' National Strategy*. London: HMSO.

Department of Health (2000) *Carers and Disabled Children Act 2000*. London: Department of Health.

Department of Health (2001a) *Carers and Disabled Children Act 2000: Policy Guidance*, London: Department of Health.

Department of Health (2001b) *The Expert Patient: A New Approach to Chronic Disease Management for the 21st Century*. London: HMSO.

Department of Health (2004) *The Carers (Equal Opportunities Act)*. London: Department of Health.

Department of Health (2005) *Carers and Disabled Children Act 2000 and The Carers (Equal Opportunities Act) Combined Policy Guidance*. London: Department of Health.

Department of Health (2006a) *Our Health, Our Care, Our Say*. London: Department of Health.

Department of Health (2006b) *Staff in the NHS 2005*. London: Department of Health, www.ic.nhs.pubs/nhsstaff, accessed 23 November 2007.

Department of Health (2007) *Departmental Report*. London: HMSO.

Edmonds, P. (2007) 'Fighting for everything': Service experiences of people affected by multiple sclerosis. *Multiple Sclerosis*, 13(5): 8.

Family Secrets (2007) I resent her for still being alive. *Times*, 14 November.

Finch, J. (1990) The politics of community care. In C. Ungerson (ed.) *Gender and Caring: Work and Welfare in Britain and Scandinavia*. New York: Harvester Wheatsheaf.

Fine, M. & Glendinning, C. (2005) Dependence, independence or inter-dependence? Revisiting the concepts of care and dependency. *Ageing and Society*, 25: 601–19.

Fisher, M. (1994) Man-made care: Community care and older male carers. *British Journal of Social Work*. 24(6): 659–80.

Forster, A. & Young, J. (1996) Specialist nurse support for patients with a stroke in the community: A randomised controlled trial. *British Medical Journal*, 312: 1642–6.

Gattuso, S. & Bevan, C. (2000) Mother, daughter, patient, nurse: Women's emotion work in aged care. *Journal of Advanced Nursing*, 31(4): 892–9.

Gaylin, W. (1985) Feelings. IK. Vaux (ed.) *Powers that Make Us Human: Foundation of Medical Ethics*. Urbana, IL: University of Illinois Press.

Geddes, J. M. L. & Chamberlain, M. A. (1994) Improving social outcome after stroke: An evaluation of the volunteer stroke scheme. *Clinical Rehabilitation*, 8: 116–26.

Griffiths Report (1988) *Community Care: An Agenda for Action; a Report to the Secretary of State for Social Services by Sir Roy Griffiths*. London: HMSO.

Heaton, J. Arskey, H. & Sloper, P. (1999) Carers' experience of hospital discharge and continuing care in the community. *Health and Social Care in the Community*, 7(2): 91–9.

Henderson, J. & Forbat, L. (2002) Relationship-based social policy: Personal and policy constructions of 'care'. *Critical Social Policy*, 22(4): 669–87.

Herring, J. (2007) Where are the carers in healthcare law and ethics? *Legal Studies*, 27(1): 51–73.

Hochschild, A. (1983) *The Managed Heart: Commercialisation of Human Feeling*. Berkeley, CA: University of California Press.

Henwood, M. (1998) *Ignored and Invisible? Carers Experience of the NHS*. London: Carers' National Association.

Hirst, M. (2001) Trends of informal care in Great Britain during the 1990s. *Health and Social Care in the Community*, 7(2): 91–9.

James, N. (1992) Care = organisation + physical labour + emotional labour, *Sociology of Health and Illness*, 14(4): 488–509.

Laverack, G. (2005) *Public Health: Power, Empowerment and Professional Practice*. Basingstoke: Macmillan.

Lloyd. L. (2000) Caring about carers: Only half the picture? *Critical Social Policy*, 20(1): 136–49.

Logan, P. A., Aham, J., Gladman, J. R. F. & Lincoln, N. B. (1997) A randomised control trial of enhanced social services occupational therapy for stroke patients. *Clinical Rehabilitation*, 11: 107–13.

May, J., Ellis-Hill, C. & Payne, S. (2001) Gatekeeping and legitimization: How informal carers' relationship with health care workers is revealed in their everyday interactions. *Journal of Advanced Nursing*, 36(3): 364–75.

Nolan, M. (2001) Supporting family carers in the UK: Overview of issues and challenges. *British Journal of Nursing*, 10(9): 608–13.

Parker, G. & Clarke, H. *(2002)* Making the ends meet: Do carers and disabled people have a common agenda? *Policy and Politics*, 30(3): 347–59.

Pickard, L. (2001) Carer break or carer blind? Policies for informal carers in the UK. *Social Policy and Administration* 35(4, September): 441–58.

Power, C., Atherton, K., Strachan, D. P., Shepherd, P., Fuller, E., Gibb, I., Kumari, M., Low, G., Macfarlane, G. J., Rahi, J., Rodgers, B. & Stansfield, S. (2007) Life-course influences on health in British adults: Effects of socio-economic position in childhood and adulthood. *International Journal of Epidemiology*, 36(3): 532–9.

Royal Commission on Long Term Care (1999) *With Respect to Old Age: Long Term Care- Rights and Responsibilities*, Cm 4192-I, London: HMSO.

SCIE (2004) *Practice Guidance to Carers (Equal Opportunities) Act*, www.carers.gov.uk.

Thompson, S. C., Bundek, N. I. & Sobolew Schubin, A. (1990) The caregivers of stroke patients: An investigation of factors associated with depression. *Journal of Applied Social Psychology*, 20: 115–29.

Tomkinson, B. (2006) I live with someone I've lost. *The Guardian*, 6 May.

Tronto, J. C. (1993) *Moral Boundaries. A Political Argument for an Ethic of Care.* New York: Routledge.

Turner, B. (1987) *Medical Power and Social Knowledge*. London: Sage.

Twigg, J. & Atkin, A. (1994) *Carers Perceived: Policy and Practice in Informal Care.* Buckingham: Open University Press.

Ward, F. (2007) Head of skills, research and intelligence at Skills for Care, cited in A. Cole, In search of the invisible workers. *The Guardian*, 17 October.

Yeandle, S., Bennett, C., Buckner, L., Fry, G. & Price, C. (2007a) *Diversity in Caring: Towards Equality for Carers*. Report No. 3. Carers, Employment and Services report series. Leeds: University of Leeds.

Yeandle, S., Bennett, C., Buckner, L., Fry, G. & Price, C. (2007b) *Stages and Transitions in the Experience of Caring*. Report No. 1. Carers, Employment and Services report series. Leeds: University of Leeds.

Afterword: Principles, Power, Professionalism and Partnership

Georgina Koubel

The authors of this book come from a range of disciplines and in several cases the chapters, and indeed the editorial process itself, have emerged from a process of collaboration between people from diverse disciplines and professional backgrounds. As such, the book contains an eclectic series of models and theoretical frameworks that practitioners can use to inform their practice. This reinforces the notion that service users can benefit from a coalition of views and perspectives, even if there are issues of difficulty and conflict, so long as the people involved can acknowledge their differences, respect the perspectives of their colleagues and, most importantly, remain person centred in their approach (Quinney 2006).

Principles

People are attracted to the fields of health and social care for a myriad of reasons, but the one given most frequently at interviews for applications to university is the desire to 'help people'. The traditional principles and values underpinning person-centred care and basic counselling skills (Nelson-Jones 2008), such as respect for individuals and unconditional positive regard, are therefore fundamental to all of the health and social care professions. This is not to say that they are always easy to put into practice. One size definitely does not and never can fit all. People who use services also come in a variety of different packages and the person-centred practitioner needs to be aware of the impact of social factors such as the age, 'race', gender, sexuality, class and (dis)ability of the person with whom they are working in order to engage with them appropriately. Not everyone in society has been enabled to engage in partnership and planning, and many of the most vulnerable people who use health and social services may have been denied opportunities to develop these skills. Equally, the previous experiences those individuals have had with professionals and other figures in authority will inform their perspectives, and any negative connotations may have been further exacerbated by the attitudes and behaviours of others towards them (Graham 2007). Obviously this will inform their ability to form a relationship of mutual trust with practitioners.

Although some professions such as social work may place higher on their list of priorities more radical notions involving citizenship and social justice, these principles are also key to the understanding and application of person-centred care. This means that all practitioners need a working knowledge of the principles of the Human Rights Act 1998 and the requirement, as Thompson and Thompson (2005: 22–3) propose, for us all to ensure that our practice reflects the intention that 'a philosophy of human rights should become part of the culture of the UK legal system and even of UK society more broadly'.

The management of competing rights or the balancing of rights with risks will continue to challenge practitioners in health and social care. Issues of choice, vulnerability, independence and safeguarding will continue to highlight areas of conflict and difference. However, these inform the most important principles within the 'caring' professions and our jobs require us to work with those conflicts while also trying to maintain positive and supportive relationships with the individuals who use services. Sometimes this means letting people take risks that we consider unwise; so long as they have the capacity to understand the consequences, the practitioner needs to step back and allow people to make their own decisions. This can be hard, but it is part of the process of giving over some of our 'professional power' to the people whose lives are directly affected by the decisions they make.

Power

It is important that the constructs and models we carry in our heads include an understanding of the impact that inequality, prejudice and discrimination can have on people who use services. We need to be attuned to the notion of diversity and recognize that images surrounding 'race', gender, age and sexuality, for example, are part of who we are as practitioners and inform the ways in which we relate to people as well as how they understand our roles and responsibilities. Power and the ability to exercise that power over people from different ethnic groups can lead to discrimination in social structures and social relations (Graham 2007). As practitioners who have the power at times to decide who gets services or how those services are delivered, we need to be aware of our own capacity for prejudice with service users and other practitioners.

There is a danger in assuming that power in itself is a bad thing. It is actually as neutral as any other concept and can only be understood in relation to its context. It is possible to conceive of power as being a positive force, otherwise why would we wish to empower service users? Empowering service users means that we have to engage with the notion of their right to have a fully developed relationship within the processes of assessment, planning and service delivery. This means being open to the idea of genuine, authentic partnership with both service users and colleagues from different backgrounds. It means moving beyond the potentially tokenistic rhetoric of 'service user involvement', on the one hand, or the uncritical assumption, on the other, that all people who use services, given adequate information, will have the ability to exercise their rights as citizens to challenge oppressive practice (Banks 2006).

Professionalism

Professional practice has a long history for many practitioners and within that history lies the presumption of not only professional expertise but also professional privilege, professional perks and professional hierarchies of knowledge. These can disempower other practioners and other people who work with professionals, never mind the value given to the perspectives of service users and carers. Many professionals spend years training to reach their goal and along the way become socialised into believing that their profession is the guardian of the most important or perfect knowledge, and that the knowledge and ideologies possessed by others are of less worth or value. Professionals can obscure their knowledge with the use of incomprehensible, technical language that alienates and undermines the role of other practitioners and service users. Many service users would like to challenge notions of specialist knowledge and expertise as belonging exclusively to professionals. Experience of long-term conditions can make the service user the expert and the professional someone who can learn from that person's experience.

Service users and carers may experience professionals as remote, unapproachable, incomprehensible and even arrogant. Working within the interprofessional team should enable diverse views and perspectives to be shared fully and frankly, with the wishes and needs of the service user held firmly at the forefront of the decisions and plans that will be made. Interprofessional collaboration depends on breaking down the professional enclaves of elitism and making them more accessible to all members of the team. The question then arises: Who is and who is not a member of the team?

Partnership

Working in health and social care means above all working with people. This book has highlighted some of the psychological strategies, organizational imperatives and sociological structures that can inhibit person-centred practice. This is not to say that there are people out there in practice deliberately choosing to do harm to others or to minimise their personhood. However, unreflective practice, practice that is unaware of the harm it can do, has the potential to damage, disable and disempower. Unless we are all conscious of the ethical and cultural frameworks that are needed to inform person-centred practice, there is a real risk that better interprofessional working could lead to increased oppression or disadvantage for service users. If professionals divided are powerful to service users, how much greater is the risk of disempowerment when they team up together to tell service users what is best for them? We need to find a different way of understanding professionalism that focuses on our obligations to service users and our determination to work together in partnership with people in a way that recognises and values the diversity of experience that people who use services bring, in the same way that we value that brought by people in our own profession as well as those from other disciplines and backgrounds.

All practitioners need to find ways within the time-strapped, resource-limited cultures that hold sway in health and social care to reflect on what they do, to think about the ways in which they do it and, most importantly, to see service users as genuine, authentic partners in the process. Critical analysis of the 'taken for granted' enables practitioners to question and try to understand why things are done as they are, and whether there could be a better way. Service user perspectives, if really valued and listened to, can provide an antidote to the kinds of managerialism and professionalism that compartmentalise and exclude the personal from the professional agenda. Thoughtful reflective practice that enables transparent and honest communication between all parties offers an opportunity for better future experiences for users of health and social care services. Person-centred practice that acknowledges, respects and values the perspectives and experiences of all contributors is the level of practice to which all practitioners should aspire. Best practice relies on good, collaborative relationships, informed by the best knowledge, skills and values that each person within the partnership can provide.

References

Banks, S. (2006) *Ethics and Values in Social Work*, 3rd edn. Basingstoke: Palgrave Macmillan.
Graham, M. (2007) *Black Issues in Social Work and Social Care*. Bristol: Policy Press.
Nelson-Jones, R. (2008) *Basic Counselling Skills: A Helper's Manual*, 2nd edn. London: Sage.
Quinney, A. (2006) *Collaborative Social Work Practice*. Exeter: Learning Matters.
Thompson, N. & Thompson, S. (2005) *Community Care*. Lyme Regis: Russell House.

Index